Respecting Patient Autonomy

Respecting Patient Autonomy

Benjamin H. Levi

University of Illinois Press
Urbana and Chicago

1 2 3 4 5 C P 5 4 3 2 1

This book is printed on acid-free paper.

Library of Congress Cataloging-in-Publication Data
Levi, Benjamin H. (Benjamin Horowitz), 1961–
Respecting patient autonomy / Benjamin H. Levi.
p.   cm.
Includes bibliographical references (p.   ) and index.
ISBN 0-252-02441-9 (cloth : acid-free paper)
ISBN 0-252-06749-5 (pbk. : acid-free paper)
1. Patient participation. 2. Autonomy (Psychology)
3. Medical care—Decision making. 4. Patient satisfaction.
I. Title.
R727.42.L48   1999
610.69'6—ddc21   98-25360
CIP

To Shaun
    for everything

To my father, Floyd R. Horowitz,
    for teaching me the meaning of autonomy

To my mother, Frances Degan Horowitz,
    for living the standards of excellence and
    professional conscientiousness I have come to value

Nothing is there to come and nothing past,
But an eternal *now* does ever last.

—Abraham Cowley

Contents

Acknowledgments

I would like to thank Nicholas Burbules, Gerald Dworkin, Walter Feinberg, Jefferson McMahon, George Geiger, and Ralph Page for the help, encouragement, and intellectual rigor they have provided me throughout the years. Each has contributed to my intellectual and philosophical development and has helped me hone my ideas and my ability to express them. I thank you deeply. I am indebted to Michael Green for his ever insightful comments and provocative feedback. I thank Elizabeth Davies, Amy Gelband Mac-Donald, Robert Sostheim, and Bobbi Schultz for their help in making my dialogues realistic and accessible. I am grateful to Martin Greenberg for his support of my work in bioethics throughout my pediatrics training. I particularly wish to thank Howard Aizenstein for endlessly (and mercilessly) sharpening my philosophical skills and Jennifer Berman for her constant friendship and support. Lastly, I would like to thank Diane Gottheil and all the people who make up the Medical Scholars Program at the University of Illinois for having created the kind of interdisciplinary intellectual community that supports and nurtures work such as mine.

① The Setup

It is a source of both great joy and consternation that nothing in life stands alone. Our ideas, our practices, in fact the vast majority of our lives are so interrelated as to make meaning and understanding depend upon our powers of integration, our ability to draw interconnections. Take, for example, the simple phenomena of lightning and thunder. One begins with just the bare perception of light and sound, then perhaps their association. But not until we form some explanation for how these phenomena operate, some explanation for their interconnections, do they acquire meaning. Modern science's explanation is that both lightning and thunder result from electrical discharges in the atmosphere, which in turn emit energy. Meteorologists explain that lightning results from this energy radiating forth as light, while thunder is due to the displacement of air molecules which then collide loudly as they rush back to fill the atmospheric vacuum that was created. The two are separated in time because sound takes about five seconds to travel a mile while light travels over nine hundred thousand times faster. Whether or not one endorses this explanation, the point is that explanations create meaning by integrating distinct events and experiences with other aspects of our lives, putting them into context by showing interconnections with other ideas and practices and values.

Over the course of this discussion I hope to provide a conception of ethics, and in particular a conception of bioethics, that is concerned with examining such interconnections. More specifically, I hope to provide a model for *doing bioethics* whose focus is helping those involved with health care become more sophisticated in their understanding of what their practices and beliefs and values mean, a model that helps people connect and integrate what goes on in health care with the broader sphere of human activity. In large part, then, I am going to argue that it makes sense to provide a model for doing bioethics that is essentially and fundamentally educational. In some ways, of course, there is nothing at all new about this approach to ethics. The tradition of understanding philosophy as education dates back easily to Aristotle and Socrates, and in this century the American pragmatist John Dewey made such a conception of philosophy his signature.

But though greater or lesser portions of the model I refer to turn up in the contemporary literature, clinical bioethics by and large are not conceived of as having education as its goal, as helping people develop a deeper understanding of the nature and meaning of what they do and believe and value.[1] As so much else in medicine, bioethics has been conceived largely as beyond the understanding of most people concerned with health care. Far from being an open forum that engages those most immediately in contact with health care, much of bioethics has become the diffusion of abstract "expert" opinion. Take as evidence the phenomenon of Derek Humphrey's best-selling book on suicide and active euthanasia, *Final Exit.* Humphrey's lay perspectives have been widely criticized by professional bioethicists as simplistic and biased. Susan Wolf of the Hastings Center has gone so far as to dub his polemic "propaganda and diatribe." In the face of an enormous bioethical literature on the subject how can the overwhelming appeal of Humphrey's book be explained? Wolf suggests that *Final Exit*'s popularity is due in no small part to the abstract, detached, and somewhat incestuous nature of bioethics: "The sad truth is that those of us in the field of bioethics may indeed have done the public a disservice." Wolf continues, "I suspect we will . . . have to intensify our efforts . . . to speak deliberately and clearly to those beyond the borders of our discipline, including real patients and families. . . . There is a growing critique of a bioethics overly driven by abstract principles from which we seem to deduce the answers to human dilemmas in a way that is sterile and empty of human experience."[2]

There are of course reasons for the detached and often exhortative style that so many approaches to doing bioethics have taken. Not only are such approaches easier to conduct but they also make it easier to reach definitive conclusions, which for many people are the driving force behind bioethics. But there is something deeply and disturbingly noneducational about exhortative approaches. For when doing medical ethics is seen simply as a mechanism for providing answers to perplexing ethical conflicts, answers generated by an "intellectual elite," the average person is not engaged. Any *real* debate or argument occurs far removed from the nurse, the patient, the pharmacist, the daughter, the physician, the respiratory therapist, the social worker, the phlebotomist, and so forth. The result is a conception of doing bioethics that is not inclusive or dialogical or empathic, but rather exclusive and didactic and often all too abstract. If we want people to be reflective and responsible (if not ethical), then we must do everything in our power to help them develop understanding and insight into the meaning of their practices and beliefs and values. I contend that the core of doing bioethics should be about education.

Before explaining in what sense my approach to bioethics should be seen as an educational model, I need to provide some parameters for the discussion. First, I do not intend to present an overarching or totalizing model attempting to show how bioethics issues, collectively, can be regarded and dealt with in an educational way. Not only is the list of possible topics endless but so is the number of educational approaches, no one of which is adequate for addressing the full breadth of issues that describe bioethics. Second, I intend to provide a model *by modeling* an educational approach. In other words, rather than simply describe what would count as an educational way of handling a particular issue, I intend for my discussion to embody and exemplify those educational features that I think should characterize the process of doing bioethics. This is a difficult conceptual task, however, for both myself and for you, the reader. For me it is difficult because for an educational model to be substantive, it must not only address real issues but also integrate relevant theoretical concerns with a wide array of practical concerns. Theoretical questions such as, How should medical decisions get made? and What role should ethical principles play? and What are the implications of respecting patients' autonomous decisions? will need to be answered in ways that adequately address the actual interpersonal and professional relationships that frame bioethics conflicts, in ways that fit the political and economic and structural realities of the medical environment. Such an integrative model is challenging for the reader in that it demands attention to the subtext. That is, the reader must look beyond the discussion itself, beyond the arguments being presented, to register and consider the educational nature of what is being expressed. I will attempt to make this task, if not easier, at least clearer by providing both an overview of the issues I will cover and a ground plan for the educational themes I hope my model will manifest.

Before doing that, however, a third parameter needs to be discussed, namely, the subject matter itself. I have chosen the matter of personal autonomy as the subject of my discussion for a number of reasons. On a personal note, a long-standing interest of mine is the proper relation between the individual and her community. There exists an uneasy balance between the individual's demand to be recognized and treated as a self-governing being and the claims of society to stipulate the conditions that license an individual to act as she sees fit. Coming to terms with this balance of forces is integral to my motivation for investigating the meaning, value, and place of personal autonomy within much of Western society. Additionally, how-ever, I believe that how we as a society understand and respect personal autonomy is central to our[3] moral system, and subsequently fundamental at a number of different levels for dealing with health care concerns. For example, at the level of the individual, which medical decision-making process we endorse will depend in large part upon our understanding and valuation of personal autonomy. At the institutional level, how different policies hinder or promote autonomy likewise influences the nature of our support for those policies. Also on a normative level, our conception of and regard for autonomy funds our beliefs about the very purpose(s) of health care and the priority that patients' wishes should be granted. Given this pervasive influence, I see great value in coming to terms with personal au-tonomy as it bears on the practice of medicine. Despite an ever-expanding literature on the subject of autonomy, there remain both substantive dis-agreements about its place and value as well as substantial misconceptions about what it actually means.[4]

My hope is that this examination of autonomy contributes to our gener-al understanding of the concept, our appreciation of its importance, and our conception of what it means to respect a person's autonomous deci-sions. But as importantly, I hope that the discussion itself can help provide an inclusive and educational model for *doing bioethics,* one that effectively integrates philosophical, educational, and practical concerns. For how we go about ethical inquiry and analysis can make an enormous difference in terms of the issues considered, emphasized, and ultimately resolved.[5]

The Ground Plan

My position on personal autonomy is fairly straightforward. Explicitly, I will analyze the concept of personal autonomy, formulate a particular concep-tion of it, defend the view that patients' autonomous decisions should be respected in all primarily self-regarding matters, and finally show how this view might play out in various medical contexts. More elusive is showing how this material comes together to reflect the educational perspective I believe should characterize doing bioethics.

That bioethics is often not educational may reflect its origins within a medical tradition that tends not to cultivate educationally minded practi-tioners. Take, for example, the training of physicians.[6] Medical schools are steeped in a culture of rote memorization. Both entrance and progress ex-ams are notorious for their failure to evidence critical thinking or approach issues from multiple perspectives. Even in the context of medical decision-making, problem-solving often takes a backseat to professional socialization, as future physicians are taught to defer to hierarchy and are rewarded for doing things the way they have always been done. One has only to look at the resistance of most medical doctors to even consider the efficacy of such well-established therapies as acupuncture or biofeedback or herbal medicine to see the resistance to move beyond accepted paradigms. Indeed, the tradition of Western medical practice is strewn with unquestioned (unquestionable?) premises and assumptions.[7] Of course, many bioethicists want to challenge such premises and assumptions. Their inquiry, however, is all too seldom a process for raising the critical awareness of the majority of those who work in medicine. Institutionally, many hospitals have rushed to create ethics committees whose business (it seems) is to formulate and hand down what will become the accepted *ethical* canon. This is not to say it is wrong to work to incorporate various ethical tenets into the policies of one's institution. But insofar as doing bioethics is conceived of primarily as a reliance on "expert" opinion, such a conception is all too impoverished. Moreover, formal bioethics discussions are commonly dominated by physicians,[8] who in addition to being but a small segment of those concerned with health care are, as a group, not very representative of society's gender, racial, and socioeconomic mix and have no special sophistication with ethical issues. Of course, many ethics committees and programs have resident bioethicists with training in philosophy, theology, religion, and other appropriate fields. Still, bioethics is commonly conceived of as something handed down by an elite *not* to develop in people a greater awareness and sophistication about their beliefs and practices and values but to create (different) rules of conduct. This may be appropriate for the law, but ethics should have much more to do with education.

In my ensuing discussion of autonomy I mean to model an educational approach in the following ways. First, I will address the definition of autonomy by exploring the components that might comprise autonomy instead of by defending an already constructed definition against counterarguments. Such an approach encourages the reader to explore for herself possible configurations for understanding what personal autonomy means and involves; it avoids forcing the reader to consider autonomy *in terms of* a given orientation. By open-endedly examining the question What is personal autonomy and why is it important? the approach pushes the reader to examine the alternatives in terms of her own beliefs and to establish her own place on the spectrum. Moreover, by using dialogues and real clinical situations as the backdrop, the approach compels the reader to critique the real life characters and practices of health care in terms of the values and goals they promote. That such a critique is a product of the reader's analysis rather than the author's is in part what differentiates this approach from those that do not take education as a primary focus. For my goal is not to arrive at a prescription for what it means to respect patients' autonomy, but to foster a deeper and more critical understanding for working through the relevant issues and conflicts. To the extent that such an understanding develops, an educational approach to bioethics enables health care providers (HCPs) to construct greater meaning within their own lives. Relatedly, such an approach also enables HCPs to better gauge patients' values, concerns, and decisions, putting them into a broader, more readily understood context.

A second major educational component of the ensuing discussion is the use of dialogue. Part of an HCP's responsibility involves seeking to understand the patient, a task that is by all accounts not trivial since between any two individuals there must remain a gap—in perception, experience, feeling, and interpretation. And if an HCP is to promote the interests of any given patient, that HCP must seek to bridge some measure of that gap and thereby gauge the meaning of the patient's utterances as well as the values and concerns contained therein. And therein lies the value, the educational value, of dialogue, because dialogue constitutes a process for overcoming separation, for achieving interconnections, for relating one's own beliefs and practices and values to those of others and to the world at large. Strategic reasons for overcoming the separation between individuals are straightforward. If as a physician I cannot connect with the patient, I cannot help her. But beyond this, such interconnections enrich the meaning of our interactions, and it is in this creation of greater meaning that dialogue functions as an educational process. Moreover, because dialogue demands a certain level of mutuality, it is a self-perpetuating educational process. For to be engaged in dialogue is to be willing to examine and work to remove barriers to greater understanding. This does not mean that for dialogue to succeed its participants must be equal in all respects. Rather, the point embedded in dialogue's mutuality is this: so long as we treat others as moral equals and we are genuinely open to confronting our ignorance, biases, and insecurities, as well as the various imbalances in power, knowledge, and experience that interfere with understanding, there is no endpoint to the level of connectedness, understanding, and thereby meaning that can develop.

Part of what I hope to show in the course of this work is that such a dialogical process for overcoming differences is altogether compatible with the roles that HCPs play and the realities of the medical environment. Additionally, I mean to show that dialogue is an appropriate and educational model for respecting the exercise of patients' autonomy insofar as dialogue promotes both mutuality and understanding *and* provides HCPs with a realistic mechanism for generating creative and meaningful interactions that deal directly with the issues at the core of respecting autonomy.

What Is All This Talk about Dialogue?

Despite the current tendency to use the term *dialogue* interchangeably with *conversation* or even *talk,* a well-established tradition in philosophy, linguistics, hermeneutics, educational theory, anthropology, literary theory, and related disciplines regards *dialogue* as something special. Examining the etymology of *dialogue,* Vincent Crapanzano writes that it is "a speech across, between, through two people. It is a passing through and a going apart. There is both a transformational dimension to dialogue and an oppositional one—an agonistic one. It is a relationship of considerable tension."[9] This tension arises out of our uniqueness as individuals with particular perspectives on and of the world. One consequence is that any time we venture beyond ourselves we encounter difference that somehow we must relate to, otherness that somehow we must come to terms with. For many who write on the subject, dialogue is an attempt to mitigate the tension of otherness by engaging individuals in a deep and unencumbered interaction, an engagement that has the potential not only to overcome undesirable barriers but also to create meaning and an enriched sense of self in the process.

Because every encounter is unique, and so too each attempt to contend with the tension of otherness, obviously it is difficult to describe, and virtually impossible to define, exactly what should count as dialogue. Still, some points can be made. Nicholas Burbules emphasizes that dialogue is a practice *grounded in* human relations: "Dialogue is not something we do or use it is a relation that we enter into."[10] On this reading, the phenomenon of dialogue has to do not with utterances or even patterns of response but with the playing out of certain kinds of relationships.[11]

If we understand dialogue as a relationship concerned with coming to terms with the distinctness of human existence, it becomes clear that certain attitudes and ways of interacting will characterize successful dialogical relationships. General dispositions include being willing and able to listen thoughtfully and attentively; being prepared "to reinterpret or translate one's own concerns in a way that makes them comprehensible to others"; being open to give and receive criticism; being willing to admit that one may be mistaken; and generally being patient and tolerant of differences.[12] To actually come to terms with otherness, it is moreover important that the participants in dialogue exhibit a certain degree of commitment, if not to each other, at least to the project of the interaction. Additionally, a level of respect and reciprocity must exist between the participants if inquiry and discussion are not to be blocked by distrust, dishonesty, or disregard. This in turn requires that participants not only *be concerned with* the matter at hand (i.e., the particular aspects of otherness being dealt with) but also at some fairly deep level *have concern for* their fellow participants. For to truly come to terms with otherness one must try to embrace it as one's own concern, and in the context of dialogue it is one's fellow participants who *represent* otherness.[13]

Clearly, there is no set method for applying the above dispositions that will make an encounter dialogical. But in contrast to other forms of interaction in which the goal (of one or more participants) might be to emote or to show off or to gain dominance, dialogical encounters do require a special form of engagement. Its participants must enter into the discourse willing to grapple with the issues at hand, to search for underlying meaning and common ground, and to persevere even when the process proves uncomfortable. So conceived, dialogue is not an offhand encounter one terminates when the going gets tough. Nor is it an attempt to manipulate or bully. It is an inclusive and flexible relational process through which individuals sincerely try to transcend otherness through the use of questions, statements, criticisms, explanations, stories, body language, jokes, even silence. This is not at all to say that dialogue, by definition, must succeed at transcending otherness. Such a fusion may prove illusory—on either a practical or a theoretical level. Consensus, agreement, even mere understanding can be extremely difficult to reach. What can be said is that an encounter qualifies as *dialogue* to the extent that it genuinely exhibits or manifests a relational process of coming to terms with otherness. This focus on procedure rather than outcome reminds us that there is value in the encounter itself, apart from its particular endpoint.

This value is in many ways a developmental one. Specifically, dialogical interactions have the potential to deepen each participant's own sense of self, to create greater understanding and appreciation of otherness, and quite possibly to enrich the relationship between the participants. Further, we cannot prejudge the developmental potential for any given dialogue. Unless we can point to the ways in which dialogue is constrained *and must remain constrained,* there is no reason to think that the development of meaning, that is, the extent of development, must be constrained. In that sense, dialogical relations offer much hope, as dialogue is itself a process for transcending barriers.

Over the course of this work I hope to show that it is just this developmental potential, along with dialogue's more strategic properties, that make dialogue an appropriate, desirable, and educational process for respecting personal autonomy. Now I am not meaning to argue that to respect personal autonomy HCPs must enter into a dialogical relationship with each and every patient. Rather, I will be claiming that it is important for HCPs to understand that their encounters with patients constitute relationships, and that in certain cases there is great value in pursuing dialogue.[14] Sometimes dialogue will prove useful in discerning whether a patient is in fact autonomous. Also, dialogue actually can help promote patients' exercise of autonomy in any number of ways. And relatedly, dialogue has the potential to overcome conflicts involving patients' autonomous wishes.

That the process of dialogue is both consistent with most patient-HCP relationships and educational in character makes it particularly appropriate for the model I mean to present for respecting personal autonomy, and more generally for doing bioethics. For dialogue encourages us to rethink our understandings of ourselves and our practices and has the potential to create greater meaning in our activities, relationships, and lives in general. Moreover, it has the potential to challenge and transcend the barriers that impede inquiry and communication and, ultimately, the resolution of conflict.

Anyone even slightly familiar with the practice of medicine has seen how imbalances in power, knowledge, or even social and professional roles can interfere with health care and in particular with respecting patients' autonomy. As a mechanism for respecting and promoting patients' autonomy and thereby advancing health care, dialogical relationships have the advantage of being inclusive as well as not prejudging an individual's level of ability. This combined with dialogue's essential fluidity allows authority to shift between interlocutors and thereby adapt to the particular needs of the situation at hand rather than be constrained by rigid designations. In fact, one of the most important lessons to be gleaned from the work that has been done on dialogue is that no perspective is objective, no judgment or communication "ideologically free." And so, while it is true that we must interpret situations and others' responses to those situations, we should beware of assuming too much, of taking for granted the accuracy of our own interpretations and the extent to which a given understanding or sense of meaning is shared. Most of us perceive the light and the sound, but the connections we draw and the meanings that result may vary considerably—at least until we have had an opportunity to come together. Dialogue keeps us on our toes, so to speak, by encouraging us to question ourselves and our understanding of the world. Through dialogue we can examine the interconnections we have drawn between the world and meaning. Dialogue is in many ways a developmental process through which we can at once come to terms with otherness and fare better in the world. How dialogical interactions actually will unfold will be fleshed out below. For now, I mean only to have provided a sense of what dialogue involves and what are its implications in the context of doing bioethics. What follows is a brief overview of the ground that I will cover in this book.

An Overview

In the body of the discussion of personal autonomy I will examine two issues. First, what does it mean for an individual, call her Sally,[15] to be autonomous, self-governing? Second, what is the value of personal autonomy (within Western society), and in particular what sort of respect is owed autonomous beings, specifically patients, when they are making primarily self-regarding (PSR) decisions? I believe it makes sense to understand most adults as autonomous beings and that to do so is both philosophically and pragmatically fruitful. To establish this I will examine the general characteristics a person must possess to qualify as autonomous and discuss the nature of *being autonomous*. In addition to laying out a philosophical foundation for what personal autonomy means, I will argue that the presumption of personal autonomy is a principal underpinning of many of our moral and social intuitions, as well as our legal and political practices and institutions. More specifically, I will argue that if we are to treat them as moral equals, whose ideas and values and aspirations we must take seriously, autonomous beings must be allowed to make their own decisions—even when they make decisions we consider to be bad or imprudent.

In the course of presenting these arguments, I will respond to two particularly troubling relationist objections. The first objection is that the social nature of human development, combined with the persistent and pervasive influence of others throughout our lives, undermines the notion that most adult human beings are in fact self-governing. The second objection is that even if individuals are autonomous they exist in a culture amongst other individuals, so it is inappropriate to regard any decision as "primarily self-regarding." Without attempting to dismiss these objections out of hand, I will contend that it is the presumption of autonomy that makes possible our conception of a moral equal and that built into this is the notion that certain decisions belong to the individual. I will contend that it is because Sally is presumed autonomous that her actions have the meaning for us that they do. The sorts of relationships we establish with Sally, how we interact with her, what we expect from her, what we conceive of as her responsibilities and her due, and even ontologically what constitutes her domain, I will contend all depend upon whether we conceive of Sally as an autonomous being. Moreover, I will attempt to defend my view against those who would override the exercise of Sally's autonomy in the interests of promoting either her well-being or her future autonomy. By providing the characterization and evaluation of personal autonomy that I do, I hope to help lay the groundwork for more fully incorporating respect for personal autonomy into the ethos of medical practice.

Moving on from this philosophical argument for the meaning of personal autonomy and its primacy in PSR matters, I will turn toward the more practical task of situating my conception of personal autonomy within the context of medicine. Specifically, I will present a dialogical model for my conception of respect for personal autonomy and explain how it may be understood as a form of specified principlism[16] that also accommodates various important feminist and relationist concerns. I will argue that concern for personal autonomy can be sensitive to the responsibilities engendered by our social interaction with others if one conceives of respect for personal autonomy as a *process* that involves entering into a relationship with someone, however brief. I will further suggest that it is not always clear what it means to respect Sally's autonomous (PSR) decisions and as such it frequently will be necessary to pursue dialogue to truly respect her autonomous decisions.

In arguing that respecting personal autonomy entails entering into a relationship, one that optimally would be dialogical, I am hoping to show how a rather principlist approach can account for the dynamics of particular relationships—on both a personal and a professional level. Clearly, no model is a panacea. But I will try to show that this conception of respect for personal autonomy, in addition to being inclusive, empathic, and educational in its orientation, easily accommodates the full personal and professional dynamics of many clinical situations/dilemmas. This includes recognizing that HCPs are (in part) defined by certain professional norms and also that the seriousness of risk to a patient's health may affect the course of the patient-HCP encounter. That said, the dialogical model I present does not directly address the institutional and structural components of ethical conflicts involving personal autonomy, and in certain respects this is a serious deficit.

I also will revisit the relationist challenge to rebut the claim that all decisions are to some extent community property. For the relationist position threatens to throw open the decision-making process to the point that *no one* is in a position to decide who may be excluded from participating. What I will suggest is that because certain kinds of situations and decisions so fundamentally and thoroughly devolve on the individual (in the present context, *the patient*), they deserve the designation *primarily self-regarding;* and in these situations it must be the (autonomous) individual alone who determines what role others should be allowed to play. My claim will be that being treated as a moral equal, as an autonomous being, *means* being allowed to determine the meaning that the relationships and interconnections in one's life should have.

The Case for Respect

The real trick, of course, is translating these ideas into practice so that in the context of patient care respecting personal autonomy means something substantive. One great difficulty with many bioethical treatises is determining how to bridge the gap between theory and practice. Authors of bioethical treatises—at least the good ones—present arguments that are finely detailed, distinctions that are complex, points that are occasionally even elegant. Moreover, they manage to neatly bracket confounding factors or at least frame them in a way that makes their effect on the eventual outcome seem inappreciable. But of course this is not how real life works. In real life people's use of language is sloppy, and it is often the unspoken premises that rescue conclusions from being confusing non sequiturs. Rather than merely relevant bystanders, in practice confounding factors—such as time constraints, miscommunication, and family dynamics—frequently are instrumental in determining a situation's outcome. Nor is it always helpful when bioethical treatises introduce clinical scenarios and discussions to show how a particular theory might play out. For we still tend to overintellectualize personal interactions, making them cleaner and clearer, but at the same time less realistic.

Obviously, I have some sympathy for intellectualized approaches, for clarifying issues and teasing out relevant distinctions. But if the conception of *ethics as education* that I argue for is to succeed, the discussion of ethics carried out here cannot be so abstract that it cannot be connected with actual day-to-day human interaction. For it is precisely this tendency to abstraction that has alienated bioethics from the people who ought to be at its center, namely HCPs and patients. What makes it difficult to provide a nonabstract bioethics model, however, is that without the abstraction, the meta-analysis, what remains can easily seem mundane, even trivial. Without the added emphasis, the phonetic markings of abstract philosophical analysis, unadorned human interaction risks appearing not only plain, but also undefined. Like diamonds in the rough, when critical issues are thoroughly embedded in background material their significance often is obscured. Moreover, attempts to work through critical issues in their natural context often result in a focus on the background instead of on the critical issues themselves.

In an effort to remedy these difficulties, I have tried to make more real the process of respecting patients' autonomous primarily self-regarding (PSR) decisions by interspersing dialogues in my discussion. In these dialogues I have tried to find a balance between unadorned human interaction and an overly intellectualized account of a process whereby HCPs attempt to respect patients' autonomous choices. Not surprisingly, at times I have swung too far to one side or the other, usually erring on the side of intellectualism. To the extent that the dialogues have achieved some balance, I am indebted to the critical and generous comments of various friends and colleagues who were kind enough to remind me that philosophical discussions usually do not break out during the transition stage of labor or on the way to a cardiac arrest or between minimum-wage employees at nursing homes who are each taking care of twelve patients, seven or eight of whom have a major physical or mental debility. Perhaps unavoidably, some of the characters in the dialogues are more articulate than the average individual. Similarly, the events that transpire are somewhat unnaturally telescoped or are at least more concentrated than often occurs in real life. Still, each dialogue is based on an actual clinical situation that either I have encountered or one of my medical colleagues has.

In these dialogues I have attempted to portray the process of respecting patients' autonomous PSR decisions. By example, I have tried to present this process as involving HCPs entering into relationships with patients and attempting to overcome otherness. I have tried to show HCPs working to understand patients and their decisions; working to educate patients; and, perhaps most importantly, working to develop a deeper sense of meaning for both themselves and their patients. For by coming to understand the meaning and implications of beliefs and values and practices, both HCPs and patients are arguably in a better position to make good health care decisions. I have tried to show the importance of going beyond the face value of patients' responses and how by engaging in dialogue HCPs can help resolve some of the conflicts that involve patients' exercise of autonomy.

Clearly, it is unrealistic to imagine that all HCPs will be concerned with respecting patients' autonomous PSR decisions, much less will manifest sufficient awareness, sensitivity, and skill to engage in this process effectively. It is similarly unrealistic to imagine that all situations will lend themselves to full-fledged dialogue. Time constraints, power imbalances, unforeseen interpersonal dynamics, and institutional policies often restrict the extent to which HCPs can engage in dialogue. Sometimes this will mean that respecting an autonomous decision will involve little more than acceding to a patient's demands. On occasion it may mean that for one reason or another it will be difficult for HCPs to respect autonomous PSR decisions at all. In their attempt to show how autonomous choices *can* be respected, the five dialogues reflect these realities. Not all the characters successfully engage in dialogue. Not all the HCPs even attempt to respect patients' autonomous PSR decisions, and those that do sometimes do not handle it well or with the sophistication one might hope. Some dialogues are cut short, just as they are in real life. Some dialogues involve strangers, others longtime friends and associates who have a more intimate knowledge of the patient's beliefs and values. I purposefully have made many of the boundaries fuzzy because life *is* fuzzy. But I believe that within each dialogue lies a model for how real HCPs can engage in the kind of process that constitutes respecting patients' autonomy.

The point, then, is to critically evaluate the dialogues, to determine which aspects of the interactions presented are precious in terms of the model being presented and which are merely background material. To aid in this process, but not to guide it (since the dialogues are intended to focus and refocus the discussion as it proceeds through the issues integral for understanding what autonomy means, why it is valuable, and what is involved in respecting a patient's autonomous PSR decisions), I present some questions for reflection in the afterword. A brief assessment of this dialogical integration, this translation of theory into practice, will constitute the final chapter of the book. For unless it is realistic for actual HCPs to embrace the proposed model, the model will have fallen short of its ultimate aim.

② Background

Within the context of medicine the term *autonomy* has become a diverse catchphrase. One hears it used to refer to someone's state of mind, degree of independence, entitlement, control, even level of education. Examples of ill-defined statements about autonomy abound in the literature on autonomy: "The imperialism and arrogance of autonomy must be bridled";[1] "From a care perspective, autonomy is dangerous because it is maximized through isolation from others";[2] as well as in everyday conversation: "There's nothing left of autonomy now that managed care controls how medicine gets practiced"; "Given how little he knows about the situation, he can't be very autonomous"; "Treatment decisions aren't autonomous if patients defer to the physician's judgment"; "She violated my autonomy by not telling me I had high blood pressure"; "Respect for autonomy has gone too far! We can't give patients everything they want." What is confusing is not just the disparate interpretations but also the lack of clarity regarding what is at issue. Is autonomy a state of being, a way of acting, or a principle?

In the ensuing chapters my goal is to provide a viable interpretation of personal autonomy for the purposes of understanding how adult patients should be treated by HCPs. To that end I will examine what makes a person autonomous, discuss the relationship between having the capacity for autonomy and acting autonomously, and attempt to defend what I take to be the importance (and primacy) of respecting a person's autonomous decisions in matters that can be called primarily self-regarding (PSR), which I will explain shortly. My aim is to show that within the context of Western culture, and the practice of medicine in particular, it makes sense to regard the vast majority of adult patients as autonomous. And I will argue that given the dynamics of the medical environment and the value we attribute to being autonomous, no one other than the autonomous individual should have final say regarding her PSR health care decisions. In that sense, my ultimate goal is to defend patients' exercise of autonomy against paternalistic affronts—as opposed to measures intended to protect (or benefit) other individuals or society at large.

Though my arguments will not depend on any particular definition of paternalism, the following characterization (whose defense cannot be undertaken here) does a better job than most at capturing the full breadth of actions we call paternalistic: "A paternalistic act is one that is primarily intended to benefit the recipient, wherein the recipient's consent or dissent is not (nor would be) an overriding consideration of the initiator."[3] One particular advantage of this characterization is that it points to paternalism's failure to accord individuals the equal respect that, other things being equal, they deserve. Thus, in addition to pointing out what is prima facie objectionable about paternalistic action, the above characterization provides some relatively natural division points for what counts as *non*-objectionable paternalism. For there are clear cases in which the intended beneficiary's wishes do *not* deserve equal respect.[4]

There are a number of reasons for focusing on paternalistic affronts to the exercise of autonomy. First, they fundamentally raise issues about the purpose of human existence and thereby compel us to articulate our view of appropriate human conduct. We will regard paternalistic encroachments upon the exercise of autonomy very differently depending on whether we take happiness or self-determination or growth or some other goal as fundamental. To formulate a response to paternalism we are required to articulate what we consider acceptable behavior and what preconditions legitimate that behavior. In this regard, the issue of paternalism directly addresses how we think a person should live her life, while also indirectly addressing what is the proper relation between an individual and her community.

Second, paternalistic affronts constitute a particularly insidious assault against the exercise of autonomy. It is more difficult to challenge those who, by definition, "have one's best interests at heart." Additionally, the line between intentions to help and intentions to subvert is often unclear. Lionel Trilling commented on this insidious character when he warned of "the dangers which lie in our most generous wishes," writing that "some paradox of our nature leads us, when once we have made our fellow men the objects of our enlightened interest, to go on to make them the objects of our pity, then of our wisdom, ultimately of our coercion."[5] Thoreau, too, knew this when he commented that if ever he should see a man coming down the road with the intention of doing him good, he should run for his life. In point of fact, there is often a non-straightforwardness about paternalism's affront to the exercise of autonomy that makes it not just hard to reckon with but also insidious, and thereby potentially very dangerous.

But perhaps the most important reason for orienting this discussion in terms of paternalism is that paternalism raises issues about what it means to respect another human being. What characteristics must a person have to merit respect? What are the different senses of respect and what are the implications of according someone respect? Of course, I cannot hope to resolve all these troubling issues or many that are connected to them. I cannot address paternalism beyond the cursory sketch I have already provided. Nor can I discuss the many different ways to understand the notion of respect. Because of length restrictions, I also cannot address adequately issues directly related to a fully developed understanding of autonomy, such as factors that reduce autonomy; because I see no nonarbitrary way of resolving other issues I cannot completely define PSR decisions. But I do hope to provide an interpretation of autonomy that is reasonable and helpful and adequately demonstrates the primacy of respecting the exercise of autonomy in PSR matters.

My views are grounded in the ontological belief that the moral equality of adult human beings rests on the presumption that adults *are* autonomous beings. This said, my views also reflect a strong political belief that, especially within the practice of medicine, a great danger lurks in not regarding individuals as autonomous. Far too many of those with power foist their values on individuals deemed "incapable of governing themselves," which makes abuse virtually inevitable. Moreover, I think the failure to treat patients as capable of governing themselves contributes to not only the increasing numbers of patients feeling unempowered but also a growing distrust and unwillingness to work toward solutions among both patients and HCPs. If we wish people to develop their own capacities and take responsibility for their lives, we must treat them as moral equals, and this will include the right to make their own health care decisions as they see fit.

Of course, philosophical discussions will not change this situation; by and large they will not empower people or create a society more respectful of individual autonomy. Instead we need educational programs, policies sensitive to people's proclivities and needs, and a restructuring of institutions so that individuals are both respected and held accountable. But if we are to foster the capacity for autonomy and protect its exercise, we must understand what we mean by autonomy and its value for us. My hope is that what follows can help lay such a groundwork and that with others' contributions we can forge a common understanding about why and in what manner autonomy should be fostered, protected, and valued.

Important to the success of this project is how our discussion is framed. In the interests of creating the right ambience, I relate the following experience from my medical school clerkship in internal medicine.

I admitted a forty-six-year-old white male, whom I will call Alan, to the hospital nine months after he had been treated for mycobacterium avium intracellulare, a pathogen that primarily infects immunosuppressed individuals, which heralded his positive HIV status. Alan had been a nursing assistant for about ten years and had done volunteer work with AIDS patients during the year prior to his admission. He came to the emergency room with a sudden and progressive three-day onset of shortness of breath, extreme fatigue, dizziness, tightness in his chest, and general malaise. Alan had no history of depression, anxiety, alcoholism, drug use, suicidal thoughts, or mental impairment. Upon examination he was alert, quite articulate, and fully aware of his condition. After completing the standard workup I asked if he would be willing to discuss his preferences for medical treatment, now and in the future. At the time we discussed his preferences there was no reason to think that Alan was in any serious or immediate danger. But the prospects are grim for someone with HIV who is showing signs of AIDS, and I thought it best to document Alan's wants when he was alert, competent, and in relatively little distress. We talked about a variety of circumstances and possible eventualities. We talked about Alan's preferences and why he had them, as well as what might be the consequences of carrying out his preferences. It was clear that the rationales for some of his preferences were based primarily on fear, and that even by his own judgment some preferences were more well grounded than others. He understood the implications of his views and stood firm by his decisions. There were three procedures that he did not want done under any conditions whatsoever: bronchoscopy, lumbar puncture (or "spinal tap"), and myelogram.[6] Additionally, Alan specified that he did not want renal dialysis, tube feeding, or artificial ventilation unless the precipitating condition was reversible. Alan did not want to discuss whether he should be resuscitated in case of cardiac or respiratory distress. He explained that he had a living will, that it was at home, and that he planned to arrange for a durable power of attorney. Alan denied having any current romantic partners. He did report that he had three adult children, but also that he was estranged from all of his family, both near and distant.

Less than three hours after our discussion, and very unexpectedly, Alan's condition rapidly deteriorated. He developed a high fever, floated in and out of consciousness, and became nauseous, confused, and lethargic. The possibility of septic meningitis was an immediate concern. Septic meningitis is a rapidly progressive infection of the spinal membranes and fluid that can cause severe brain damage and death within hours if not treated immediately and properly. Because different pathogens require specific interventions and because it is especially problematic to accurately predict which pathogens have taken hold in an immunosuppressed patient such as Alan, appropriate diagnosis and treatment of meningitis requires performing a lumbar puncture. The second-year resident in charge of the case, Dr. J., knew Alan from the clinic and had overseen Alan's care in the nine months since his HIV diagnosis. Though Dr. J. believed I had accurately documented Alan's preferences and that Alan was competent and well-informed when he made his decisions regarding treatment, Dr. J. believed that performing a lumbar puncture to rule out meningitis was the right thing to do.

In one sense, no more need be said about the specifics of this case. The dilemma is straightforward: does one respect Alan's preferences or instead act paternalistically and override them? On the other hand, it is instructive to finish the story to understand how these dilemmas are often played out. While Alan remained in a stuporous condition a succession of four physicians attempted for approximately half an hour to persuade Alan of the importance of the lumbar puncture. He was asked numerous times whether he would allow the procedure. When he could be roused to answer, he said "no." At the close of the last consultation with him a physician asked if Alan did not want the doctors to do what they could to help him. When again roused to answer he replied, "I guess so." We left the room and in the ensuing discussion everyone admitted that Alan's state of mind was problematic at best and that his closing assertion would be difficult to take as an indication of much of anything. The ethical dilemma was duly recognized and discussed, and then a lumbar puncture was performed. The spinal fluid was normal, Alan recovered from his immediate infirmity, and he later said that it was "probably OK" for Dr. J. to have performed the procedure.

If anything is clear from this example it is perhaps that the same course of events can be viewed by some as entirely justified and by others as horrendously misguided. Such difference of opinion likely stems from disagreements over either of two considerations. The first consideration is to what extent various factors influence the autonomous nature (or what is sometimes called the authenticity or genuineness) of a patient's decision. Though it is impossible to provide a complete list of such factors, among them would be the setting for a patient's decision; in our case one might take into consideration the effects of being in a hospital or the stress of illness. Other influences include an agent's knowledge base or ignorance, weakness of will, fear, prudence, consistency regarding beliefs and values, impulsiveness, and the apparent rationality of a decision. Which influences are recognized as playing a role and how much weight they are given will vary from person to person. The point is that different judgments about the justifiability of paternalistically overriding a patient's decision often can be explained by different interpretations of how the circumstances of the situation affect her decision-making. Thus someone might justify Dr. J.'s action by explaining that the authenticity of Alan's decision was diminished by his "irrational" fear of a minor procedure, the stress of his immediate illness, or perhaps a general depression about his future demise. This is one approach to defending paternalistic action, to call into question the legitimacy, the genuineness of a patient's decision. As such, it involves deciding which autonomy-reducing influences are operative at a given time and the extent of their influence. Reasonable people will differ about what counts as an autonomy-reducing factor and likewise will differ in their estimations of the effect of each factor. Depending on one's assessment, one will or will not view paternalistic intervention as a legitimate option.

The second consideration is perhaps more fundamentally divisive. Here the issue is not Alan's state of mind, whether he is capable or competent to make a decision regarding his own life plan, for the doctors agree that he is competent, that his decisions are autonomous. Rather the elemental question is whether it is justifiable to override a patient's autonomous decision for his own well-being. Dr. J. readily admitted that Alan was competent and rational when he voiced his preferences, that Alan was clear about his preferences, and that Alan was able to distinguish between kinds of care and to graduate his own preferences for treatment. Moreover, Dr. J. recognized that Alan's decision was not the result of factual misconceptions. Alan was familiar with the medical profession through his work as a nurse's aid and his experiences as a patient. He had worked extensively with AIDS patients and so understood the likely course of his illness. And finally Alan had been pressed (by myself) to seriously consider the implications and possible ramifications of his decisions regarding treatment. In the first consideration the issue was to determine the extent to which Alan's decision was autonomous. Here, in contrast, the question is whether the belief (or perhaps the fact) that Alan's best interests are not served by his decision makes it acceptable to override his informed autonomous decision. Here, as with the first consideration, people will differ in their views, but for many *this* difference will constitute a fundamental philosophic position about the way they regard persons and about the way they view the ultimate ends of life. I am not suggesting that different views regarding this second consideration will divide people forever and beyond all things, but that the distinction is fundamental to the way many of us think about and deal with people.

As a society, of course, we express conflicting views about the priority of well-being vis-à-vis the exercise of autonomy. Accepted paternalistic interventions include requiring motorists to wear seatbelts, prohibiting the use of certain recreational drugs, outlawing gambling, and legislating against prostitution. As yet unsettled is the legitimacy of paternalistic interventions designed to prohibit unnecessary health care procedures, fireworks, military combat for women, and tobacco. Clearly, not all these conflicts between paternalism and the exercise of autonomy are as stark, compelling, or as easily identifiable as the conflict illustrated in Alan's case. But the question of whether people should be allowed to "make their own decisions" is no less controversial or contentious when it arises in day-to-day intercourse, as it does throughout our public and private lives.

Obviously, not all decisions are open to such challenges,[7] nor do all challenges strictly concern a person's best interest. Often paternalistic concerns are wrapped up with concerns for public safety or standards of morality or even self-interest in the sense of control or personal gain. This is part of what makes Alan's case so extreme. Most instances of conflict between the exercise of autonomy and paternalism are not nearly so clear-cut or so dire and intractable. Often we must guess at a person's preferences or about her knowledgeability or even about likely outcomes. Many conflicts do not involve the contractual obligation implied by the legal liability that attends medical care. Most people are not as estranged from family and other social relationships as was Alan. Thus, for most people life decisions take on more of an "other-regarding" character than they did for Alan. Also few can act with the prescience of their future as can someone with AIDS, whose prognosis is often grim and whose demise is often rapid and predictable. But these particulars do not make Alan's situation qualitatively different from many subtler conflicts between paternalism and respecting autonomous decisions; what they do is isolate certain issues and illustrate the conflicts more clearly. But just what do we mean by autonomy, and what place does it have in our value system?

Issues in Autonomy

The term *autonomy* is etymologically rooted in the Greek city-state. By being able to impose self (*autos*) rule or law (*nomos*) city-states were regarded as self-governing bodies. This notion of autonomy as self-governance has been extended to persons through a variety of historical and political extrapolations. Politically as well as philosophically, this transition has been used to demarcate public versus private spheres of action and authority. By the midseventeenth century the individual, in general, was viewed as the fundamental unit of society, a distinct and self-determining entity whose will was regarded as his seat of government. Philosophically, this generated a number of difficulties. For while one can easily determine which government hands down the laws for a given city-state, there is no similarly clear psychological separation with regard to the individual. It is problematic to specifically identify what initiates and governs the actions or thoughts of an individual. Nonetheless, embedded in Western culture is this notion that individuals possess a single sovereign seat of self-government, generally articulated in terms of a self-governing will.[8] While contemporary authors do not entirely deny the plausibility of the concept of *will*, many reject its feasibility as *the* seat of self-government. Part of this rejection is due to the will's historical articulation by Kant and others as a noumenal entity, unconnected physically and causally from the human brain. But there are other problems. We know that children as well as many animals have quite strong wills, strong senses of what they want to do. And yet to think of such instances of will as the foundation of self-government is to confuse desire, intention, or drive with self-government. A similar problem arises with adults who act, say, during a period of depression in ways that are by their own reckoning not just out of character but foreign. It would be odd to deny that they had willed their behavior. Yet to think of it as autonomous in the sense of self-governing is to trivialize the meaning of acting autonomously. Another reason for abandoning the belief that the will is the seat of autonomy is that it implies a separation or isolation of decision-making from acculturated habits and other nonconscious behavior that is arguably representative of autonomous preferences and values. This kind of separation is not necessarily the case, but again, it is part of the tradition of positing the will as the seat of autonomy. Perhaps it makes most sense to speak of the will metaphorically as a decision-making process that is regarded as autonomous when it operates in a certain sort of way. What that way is, of course, is the $64 question.

Clearly the difficulties I have just mentioned do not all abate simply by backing off the claim for a self-determining will to some more broad-based notion of individual governance. There remains the problem of socialization. Individuals do not create themselves in a social vacuum, nor is individual development solely a matter of consciously choosing and incorporating desired traits and values. Because we are in such large measure products of our environment it is difficult to say that we are indeed *self-governing*. The philosophic difficulty has been in locating just what makes a decision or an action autonomous in a way that warrants special consideration. That is, if we want to accord special status to an act because it is genuinely a person's own, then it needs to be shown not only why it merits that special status but also in what sense it is genuinely hers, that is, autonomous. One solution to this problem is to characterize autonomy as a diachronic property, to conceive of autonomy as a capacity possessed over time. For synchronic views that look to particular decisions for the locus of autonomy tend to beg the question of whether the characteristics that frame and influence that particular decision are in fact authentic, autonomous. Still, as we will see, it is difficult using either view to discern exactly what should or should not count as autonomous behavior.

In part what is sought is some characterization of an individual, Sally, that allows us to attribute authorship rather than simple intentionality to her decisions and actions. We say that something is *intentional* if Sally meant it, in the sense that rather than being an accident or something forced on her she intended it. But suppose Sally runs "out of fear" or limps "because of pain"; we may describe her gait as intentionally undertaken and yet still not autonomous. That is, we might say that fear made her run or pain made her limp. Although to refer to fear or pain as an agent is merely a figure of speech, it is indicative of how we philosophically distinguish between various kinds of behavior—those undertaken autonomously and those not undertaken autonomously. Authorship of an act connotes more than physical responsibility, more than a desire to do it, more than intentionality. It connotes that the entity that is "most truly" Sally would endorse that action if given an opportunity to do so. This "true Sally" may have a long temporal history or may be more newly formed. What makes up such a core self (if there is any one such core self) and how we determine when it is operative (has endorsed a given decision or action) remains to be seen. But the importance of the determination should not be underestimated. For whether we consider Sally to be the author of her decisions and actions will have important implications for the sorts of relationships we form with her and the extent to which we feel justified in interfering with her life. I think it is fair to say that our judgment on this matter will drastically alter our views about how we should interact with Sally, what we should expect from her, what is her due, what are her responsibilities, and, ontologically, what constitutes *her* domain. Were it shown that Sally was *not* the author of her behavior, that her behavior was not autonomous, then we would have to rethink not only the meaning of her behavior but also our reactions to it. In point of fact, it is just this capacity for authorship that makes it possible to regard Sally as a moral equal, as someone whose beliefs and decisions must be taken seriously.

Clearly, then, in addition to its moral relevance, whether Sally qualifies as autonomous has important political implications for how decisions get made and who makes them. For when individuals (and certain kinds of decisions and behavior) are judged *non*-autonomous, they are not simply denied a certain respectability; decision-making power often is given over to others. Thus one's autonomous status is important for demarcating certain political boundaries between persons. In a sense, being recognized as autonomous gets one into the game as a player rather than as just a shareholder. And it is precisely because being regarded as autonomous is a necessary condition for being treated with equal respect—certainly morally and in many cases politically—that the burden of proof must rest with those who would deny individuals equal respect by challenging their status as autonomous beings.

Traditions of Autonomy

Since the modern age philosophers have recognized this passport function of being considered autonomous, albeit in very different ways and generally as inseparable from the concepts of freedom and liberty. They have argued, or assumed, that human beings are autonomous and that it is this fundamental capacity to be self-governing that makes possible the characteristically human forms of social, political, and ethical interaction. Even Hobbes, who denied the existence of anything in humans to which we could apply the term *will* and endorsed a particularly mechanistic account of human existence,[9] psychologically and politically was committed to the view that humans are free to decide what they want to do and at liberty to carry out their intentions.[10] Sharing Hobbes's determinism Spinoza went a step further, explicitly asserting that if we rationally understand the passions that drive us we are self-determining.[11] One sees in Locke's work the importance of the capacity for self-determination, the role played by experience, reflection, and contemplation in originating human activity. But it was not until Kant that this reliance on autonomous action was fully acknowledged and developed, not until Kant argued that a moral life (which we all have a duty to live) involves willing for oneself those rules that could be raised to universal law. Mill completed the classical formulation of autonomy by arguing that an autonomous existence was not the logical consequence of a person's rationality as Kant had thought but, instead, an ideal, a trait to be developed, and that an autonomous life is necessary[12] for achieving the greatest happiness.

Of course, these philosophers conceived of autonomy in quite different ways. They agreed on little else than that being autonomous entails a dis-

tinct, objectively determinable, self-governing entity, assumptions that have
been called into question by contemporary philosophers. Thomas Hill helps
us toward a clearer conception of what being autonomous involves by drawing a distinction between the psychological condition of self-government
and autonomy as a right.[13] Arguing for a more complex set of distinctions,
Joel Feinberg has identified four distinct (albeit related) senses of autonomy: the capacity to govern oneself, the actual condition of self-government,
the ideal virtue derived from that conception, and the sovereign authority
to govern oneself.[14]

Of Feinberg's four conceptions, autonomy as an ideal stands out as a the-
oretically driven concept based on a conjecture of what it might mean to be
entirely self-governing. As such, it is not of central concern. For while attempts to formulate such an ideal may help us better understand the meaning and importance we attach to self-government, and perhaps even provide
us with inspiration, when we ask what it means for a person to be autonomous, what we are after is our own standing, that is, the "normal condition."[15] We want to know what conditions Sally must satisfy for us to regard
her and treat her as an autonomous being. At base, autonomy is a concept
of and about real people, and judgments regarding its presence or absence
make a real moral and political difference in the lives of individuals.

Autonomy versus Freedom

It is perhaps useful to begin with what autonomy is not. Though autonomy often has been comingled with the more easily identified notions of
freedom or liberty, the mere absence of obstacles or even coercion does not
yield autonomy.[16] In terms of discrete actions (or decisions), we consider
Sally to have acted freely when we believe not only that it was possible for
her to have acted otherwise under the same conditions but also that it would
have been reasonable to expect Sally to act otherwise had she so chosen.[17]
In other words, freedom of action involves two elements: a three-place relation, which means that Sally is free to do X in relation to some possible
frustrating condition,[18] and a normative judgment, namely that it is not
unreasonable to expect Sally to do X despite the frustrating conditions that
exist. The importance of the normative aspect of freedom is that it allows
us to go beyond a strict logical possibility in describing someone as free or
unfree and to talk about different degrees of freedom. It allows us to explain that "your money or your life" is a paradigm for *un*freedom, not because it is impossible to act otherwise but because the situation does not
offer a *viable* option.[19]

Autonomous action, like freedom, also involves a normative element insofar as some of its constituent concepts (e.g., noncompelled action or rationality) entail value judgments. As with freedom, autonomous action also presupposes a distinct and identifiable Sally. But unlike freedom, autonomous action does not arise out of a strict three-place relation; rather, it has to do with the integrity of Sally as the source for her behavior. This is not to say that freedom and autonomy are entirely unconnected. Clearly certain kinds of unfreedom may undermine the autonomous nature of a given action, if not the agent herself.[20] But the two are distinct. As an example of freedom without autonomy simply imagine a three year old out wandering on the beach unaccompanied or a pathologically compulsive person who is sufficiently powerful for her behavior to go unchallenged or an animal in the wild. While their actions may be free, they do not qualify as autonomous. For action that is autonomous but not free imagine that Sally autonomously chooses some medical treatment not knowing that it would have been forced on her had she chosen otherwise. While the external conditions (that the treatment would have been forced on her) make her actions unfree, they affect neither the autonomous nature of her choice nor her status as an autonomous being. In the normal course of events the extent to which a person is free may bear on the autonomy of her actions, and perhaps even her general state of being. But we need to recognize that whether an action is autonomous has to do with the process by which it is made, and whether a person is autonomous at base has to do with the characteristics that person possesses.

Before we turn toward an examination of these characteristics consider the following clinical scenario. In it we see a relatively straightforward set of presumably autonomous concerns and preferences, as well as an attempt to respect the exercise of autonomy. Note that what is at issue is as much about understanding the patient as about acting in accordance with her preferences.

Dialogue 1: An Exception to the Norm

In St. Jude's emergency room most patients are treated on a first-come first-served basis. After an initial interview (and perhaps the initiation of treatment) by a registered nurse, each patient's name, presenting condition, room, and time of arrival are listed in erasable marker on a large memo board. One of the emergency department physicians then signs up for, examines, and treats each patient. Because St. Jude's is a teaching hospital, some patients are examined and treated by medical residents or by third- and fourth-year medical students, but always in conjunction with a licensed physician. Though many of the patients seen in St. Jude's emergency room have "family physicians," it is seldom the case that their physician is present in the emergency room. Hence, most patients have no previous relationship with the emergency department staff before arriving at St. Jude's.

One Friday evening Brad Aiyam, a fourth-year medical student on an elective rotation in St. Jude's emergency department, enters an exam room where Tammy Carlson has been waiting for about five minutes. Tammy is a twenty-three-year-old, white, moderately overweight female whose chief complaint is diffuse lower abdominal pain that has been getting worse over the past two weeks. Physically, Tammy does not appear to be in any obvious distress. Having no private insurance, Tammy is classified on her chart as a "public aid" patient. Brad is a twenty-eight-year-old, white, well-groomed, athletic-looking male who has been at work for about seven hours and plans to go home to his wife and child in another three hours.

BRAD: Hello, Ms. Carlson. How are you?

TAMMY: I've been better.

BRAD: Well, we'll certainly do what we can to help you. My name is Brad; I'm one of the medical students here. I've been asked to speak with you, examine you, and then I plan to speak with one of the physicians and the two of us will come back together. Is that alright with you?

TAMMY: Yeah, sure.

BRAD: Well, tell me, what's been troubling you? It says here that you've been having some pain in your abdomen for the last couple of weeks.

TAMMY: Uh-huh. It's this pulling, grabbing pain that goes almost all the way across my belly, just above my waist. I've also been feeling nauseous in the morning for the last couple of weeks and have had chills on and off for the last few days.

BRAD: Is there anything that makes the pain in your belly better or worse, like food, lying down, sitting forward, having a bowel movement, time of day, stuff like that?

TAMMY: It's worse with activity. Any time I move it just hurts.

BRAD: You say it's a pulling, grabbing pain. How long does it last, and how bad is it? I mean, if ten is the worst pain you've ever had and zero is no pain at all, what would this pain be?

TAMMY: Oh, I'd say seven or eight. And it's there all the time. Though, like I said, it gets lots worse when I try to do anything, like move or somethin'.

BRAD: Have you had any trauma to that area recently or had any pain like this before?

TAMMY: I haven't had any trauma that I know of. I did have pain like this . . . oh, about two years ago. They treated me here at St. Jude's, said I had an infection in my fallopian tubes.

BRAD: OK, well, that's certainly something we can look into, see whether that's somethin' that's going on again. There are a number of other things I'd like to follow up on, though. First, when was your last menstrual period, and was it normal for you?

TAMMY: Today's Friday. I just finished on Monday. So, I guess that's four days ago, and I didn't have any trouble.

BRAD: No unusual bleeding, pain, discharge, cramping . . . ?

TAMMY: Nope.

BRAD: Is there any chance you're pregnant?

TAMMY: No, I haven't been with anyone in a long time, and anyway, I'm on the pill.

BRAD: Have you ever been pregnant before?

TAMMY: Twice.

BRAD: Did you carry either or both of them to term?

TAMMY: No. (*Looking annoyed and suspicious, Tammy squints and squares herself to Brad.*)

BRAD: Have you had any change in your diet or traveled outside the region? Noticed any changes in your urinary habits—pain or burning when you pee, increased frequency, any signs of blood? Any changes in your bowel habits—diarrhea, constipation, black tarry stools, blood?

TAMMY: Not that I've noticed, really.

BRAD: Other than your birth control pills, are you taking any medications? Prescription, over-the-counter, any recreational drugs?

TAMMY: I use a puffer for my asthma, but nothin' else.

BRAD: Do you have any medical allergies that you know of? Bad reactions to penicillin, codeine, antibiotics, stuff like that?

TAMMY: Um, not that I know of.

BRAD: Is there anything else that I haven't asked you about, any symptoms, past medical problems, or anything that's been going on with you, bothering you, that you think is relevant or that you just want to tell me?

TAMMY: Well, I do get headaches, but that's not really anything new.

BRAD: OK. Well, I need to do a quick physical exam here, and then I'll let you know where we are.

(*In the course of a five-minute general physical exam Brad finds no abnormalities other than a mildly and diffusely tender lower abdomen.*)

BRAD: Well, my feeling is that other than the tenderness in your abdomen, I'm not finding anything out of the ordinary. Your heart and lungs sound fine; you don't seem to have any immediate signs of infection; your temperature and blood pressure are normal; there's no radiation of pain that would make me think that we're dealing with a spinal or neurological problem. What you report is fairly consistent with some sort of infectious process. I'm thinking that we ought to take some blood, look at your electrolytes, test for pregnancy just in case, and get some urine to check for any signs of a urinary tract infection. We probably also ought to go ahead and do a pelvic exam, given both the nature of your pain and your history from a couple of years ago . . .

TAMMY: Someone else is gonna be here for the pelvic exam, right?

BRAD: Absolutely. There's always a nurse in the room no matter what. Now, I'm planning on going to speak with one of the physicians, getting these tests ordered, and then the two of us will come back, and he'll probably ask you some of the same things I have. Does that sound alright to you?

TAMMY: Uh, yeah.

BRAD: Now, obviously, you want to get to the root of the pain you're having. But other than that, is there anything in particular you're concerned about? Anything you want us to specifically check for or let you know about? Any questions you have for me right now?

TAMMY: Not really.

BRAD: OK. We'll be back in about five or ten minutes.

(*After speaking with Dr. Norm Rios and communicating what has transpired, Brad orders the tests, tells Tammy's nurse, Joanne, that they need to do a pelvic exam, and asks if Joanne would get everything ready. About ten minutes later, after Tammy has provided some urine and had blood taken, Brad and Norm return to the room where Joanne has prepared Tammy for a pelvic exam. Tammy is quietly sitting up on the exam table awaiting instructions.*)

NORM: Hello Tammy, I'm Dr. Rios, one of the physicians here. Brad's told me about the problems you've been having, and I agreed we ought to run those lab tests. Can you tell me a little bit about your previous infection in your fallopian tubes?

TAMMY: It's pretty much like I told him. About two years ago I got this infection that the doctor said was in my fallopian tubes and . . .

NORM: Was it on both sides, do you know?

TAMMY: I think so.

NORM: How was it treated and did it resolve alright?

TAMMY: I guess so. I took some antibiotics. And so did my husband. But I'm not married to him anymore. And I haven't had any problems since.

NORM: OK. Well, like Brad told you, we really ought to do a pelvic exam to make sure it's not the same kind of infection again.

TAMMY: Is he gonna do it or are you?

NORM: Brad's very good at these. I'm going to repeat one part of the exam just to make sure. But Brad's a real pro. (*As Brad and Norm each start to put on rubber gloves, Tammy's discomfort with the situation becomes increasingly obvious. In an attempt to break the tension, Norm tries to joke with Tammy.*) You act like you don't enjoy these things. I thought everyone liked having these done. Joanne, you always enjoy it, don't you?

(*Joanne laughs a bit nervously, but doesn't say anything.*)

TAMMY: No offense intended, but I don't . . . I just don't like the idea of him practicing on me.

BRAD: Well look, obviously, Ms. Carlson, this decision is up to you, and I won't take offense if you decide . . .

NORM: Miss Carlson, this is a teaching hospital. Student doctor Aiyam has already had a great deal of training, and you should realize that patients in teaching hospitals get better care precisely because of the students. Dr. Aiyam has done lots of these, and I'm sure if you knew how good he is, you wouldn't have any objections.

TAMMY: (*As Tammy continues to protest her tone becomes increasingly heated.*) Look, I came in here because I'm sick, not to give someone practice. I don't need to be patronized. I know that the reason I'm getting treated this way is because I'm on public aid. If I were some rich woman you know I wouldn't be gettin' practiced on.

BRAD: Um, before this goes much further, Ms. Carlson . . . as far as I'm concerned, if you would rather have Dr. Rios do this exam I really don't have any problem with that. But I get the sense that there's something else bothering you . . .

TAMMY: I don't like being patronized and (*referring to Dr. Rios*) I don't want *him* touching me either.

NORM: (*impatiently and looking for a quick exit*) I've got some other patients I need to see. Brad, when you get this sorted out have Joanne come get me if you need.

(*There is an awkward silence after Dr. Rios leaves the room. Joanne remains, waiting.*)

BRAD: Um, obviously, this whole thing must be getting pretty uncomfortable for you. I've never had one myself, but I'm told that pelvic exams aren't any fun to begin with. So I'm sure it doesn't help to have these dynamics on top of that. But I'm getting the sense that there's something else, something about this whole business that's bothering you. Are there, um . . . have you had particularly bad experiences in the past that are related to what's going on here?

JOANNE: Uh, if you'll excuse me. When y'all are ready, Brad, just come get me. I'll be doing some things just down the hall.

BRAD: OK. Thanks, Joanne.

(*Again, there is an awkward silence.*)

BRAD: Is there something in particular that's sort of, um, behind your feelings here?

TAMMY: Look, I really don't mean you any offense. But I've seen what happens when somethin' goes wrong. *You're* the one that gets hurt, and the doctor gets to walk away. And I just want to keep my chances for gettin' hurt low, if you know what I mean.

BRAD: I guess I'm a little confused here. What sort of hurt are you thinking of?

TAMMY: My sister was havin' a baby and she wanted to have it the regular way. And they made her have a, whaddaya call it, a c-section. And there was someone who wasn't a full doctor, and my sister had the baby alright, but now she can't have any more kids. I don't want that happenin' to me. I've already had two miscarriages. I don't need anyone messin' anything up more. I mean, I don't know you from Adam. And the way they treat people who don't have any money . . . well, let's just say you gotta look out for yourself around here.

BRAD: Well, everything you said is all fair enough. I can't speak for your sister's situation, but given that experience I can see why you feel the way you do. Before I say anything else, though, let me say that from a medical standpoint it's pretty important that you have a pelvic exam done, especially given your previous infection. But if you don't want me to be the one to do it, I really don't have any problem with that. Not only do I think patients should have final say, but also it's starting to sound like you have some particular concerns about your present condition that an experienced physician might be better prepared to answer. That said, I think we're looking at a real different situation from your sister's. Though from a personal standpoint a pelvic exam is pretty invasive, the only thing we're planning on doing tonight is looking to make sure that there are no obvious signs of infection or structural abnormalities, using a swab to take some cultures to check for gonorrhea and chlamydia, and doing a bimanual exam so that we can actually feel for any unusual masses or areas of tenderness. And that's basically it. In terms of your being a public aid patient, to be honest, I do notice it when I look at the chart. But beyond that I don't pay much attention to it. I know some physicians take a different attitude toward public aid patients, but it's really rare that I've seen it make any difference in how the patients actually get treated. The physicians down here in the ER are on a salary from the hospital, so your insurance status really doesn't make much of a direct difference to them. And I can assure you, I don't make anything at all—in fact, I have to pay money to work here. So, while I understand your apprehension and your suspicions, I don't think you're really at much risk for the sorts of things you're concerned about.

TAMMY: Well, maybe. But this is the only body I got. You may be different, but I've seen the way doctors look at you when you got no money. It's like they think you're less responsible 'cause you're poor, like the reason you get sick is because you don't know how to live right. And it's not like y'all explain things either. Would you have taken the time to tell me all what you did if I hadn't made a fuss? I don't know what y'all were plannin' on doin'. Y'all breeze in and breeze out, and it's not 'til someone threatens a lawsuit or somethin' that you even look up.

BRAD: Again, I can't speak for everyone in medicine, nor would I want to. But, I mean, I did ask you whether you had any questions or whether you had any specific concerns. And you said "no." Things get pretty busy here in the ER, and if I provide the opportunity and you don't take it, I just don't have time to sit down and find out if there's something you *really* want to say but haven't. It seems to me that, like anywhere else, people have to take some initiative, if you know what I mean.

TAMMY: Look, people say stuff all the time they don't mean. You got power and I got none. How am I supposed to know that you actually want to know what I think? The only way I have power for sure is by saying "no." And if I get to feelin' funny about somethin', that's what I'm gonna do, just say "no." Know what I mean?

BRAD: I guess I do. But to be honest, it seems pretty counterproductive. I mean, if you walk around assuming that everyone's out to get you, then not only can't you trust anyone, but you're not gonna be able to take advantage of what people have to offer. Take this conversation for instance. If you hadn't decided to trust me, you probably would still be angry and frustrated, and you might have even left without getting good health care.

TAMMY: (*half-jokingly*) Who says I trust you?

BRAD: Well, but I mean you sort of have to, don't you? Unless you're gonna go to medical school yourself, you have to trust someone, whether it's me or Dr. Rios or whoever. The whole system of medicine at some point depends on *you* trusting *our* judgment.

TAMMY: It may look different from your side of the fence. But from over here I don't see a whole lot to trust. You seem like you care. But most doctors I've met seem more interested in making their money and getting out on the golf course. People like me don't matter much. Ya can't have it both ways. The way doctors are anymore doesn't exactly inspire trust.

BRAD: Well, personally, I shoot pool. And other than putt-putt, I don't think I've played an actual round of golf in my whole life. But you know, it's not as if physicians have that much control—at least not the kind of control you're implying. You wouldn't believe the rules and guidelines that you have to follow, and with cost containment and all that you just don't have time to sit and talk with patients. I have that luxury, but only because I'm a medical student, and even then I probably take more time than most. And also, you gotta remember that if you're a doc, you can't turn around without worrying about a lawsuit. I know physicians who have gotten sued by patients they've never even met! I don't know . . . I think it's much more of a two-way street than you're suggesting. But anyway, now you got me goin', and I'm sure you're not interested in my personal views about how medicine ought to be. Also, I probably ought to get movin' one way or another. So how do you feel? You really should have a pelvic exam done. I'm happy to have Dr. Rios do it if you'd rather . . .

TAMMY: I guess I'd just as soon have you do it as him. But I do want that nurse here.

BRAD: You bet. I want to make sure, though . . . I don't want you to feel uncomfortable about this. But if it really is alright with you, then I'll go ahead and do the exam once I get Joanne and Dr. Rios.

(*Brad waits for a response, but Tammy doesn't say anything.*)

BRAD: OK. Before I go get them, do you have any questions or anything you want to discuss? One last chance.

TAMMY: Um, not really.

BRAD: You sure?

③ Characterizing Autonomy

General Aspects

In the preceding scenario, it was assumed that Tammy was an autonomous being (and so, too, Brad). But what are the characteristics a person must possess to be considered autonomous? Certainly basic to the concept of autonomy is *continuity of the self,* for without substantial psychological overlap in terms of memory, beliefs, habits, and feelings, it is hard to imagine in what sense one could be called "self-governing." A self is not unchanging, of course. But neither can it be so transitory that it is unconnected from moment to moment. In part, it is just such discontinuity that makes various organic brain syndromes so problematic in terms of assessing autonomy, and so tragic from a human standpoint.

Further discussion of continuity of the self risks invoking a full-blown examination of personhood, something I wish to avoid. Nonetheless, it is worth taking a moment to consider the importance for our discussion of the distinction between identity and psychological connectedness that has been made by Derek Parfit. Roughly, Parfit argues that both metaphysically and morally personhood should not be conceived of in terms of physical identity or temporal proximity, but rather in terms of psychological connectedness and continuity.[1] Arguing from a reductionist position,[2] Parfit challenges the primacy of our concern with distinct individual identity. What Parfit questions is the depth of unity for each life and the extent to which we should distinguish between different lives. That is, given the discontinuity across our own lives over time (attitudes, beliefs, awareness) and the extensive interrelationships we have with others, Parfit asks us to consider whether individual lives are not less distinct, more connected, than we normally think. Parfit's point is more than the simple observation that we are all interconnected, it is that we need to rethink the very distinctions regarding personhood upon which we base our ethical and political beliefs. If Parfit is correct, an implication for the present discussion is that we must be careful not to gloss over assumptions about distinct personhood, and that at some point we must reconcile the intimate relationship between an autonomous individual and past selves, other selves, even society at large. I will touch upon this issue below when discussing PSR actions and future selves.

A second characteristic a person must possess to be regarded as autonomous is *rationality,* that is, the ability to deliberate, analyze, and make decisions in accordance with certain rational precepts. As Joel Feinberg writes, "all those who have argued for a natural sovereign autonomy have agreed that persons have the right of self-government if and only if they have the capacity for self-government. That capacity in turn is determined by the ability to make rational choices."[3]

Of course, this criterion is not without its own difficulty. For it is not entirely clear how genuine self-governance can coexist alongside rationality's prescription to follow certain logical rules of inference, be predisposed to truth over falsehood, prefer consistency over randomness, and so forth.[4] Perhaps the way to deal with this tension is to note that, generally speaking, rationality is a designation conferred on individuals who exceed some minimum threshold of certain qualities, such as intelligence and deliberateness. Thus we might concede that certain laws of reason indeed constitute the standard for rationality, but recognize that this standard does not define rationality so much as help us identify different levels of functioning or decision-making beyond some normative threshold.

Substantively, rationality is a difficult concept to describe without remainder, but its core notion involves two major components, one normative, the other procedural. Normatively, to qualify as "rational" a person must embrace some intersubjectively accepted set of goods, what John Rawls calls primary goods. The assumption here is that a certain set of primary goods, for example, certain powers and opportunities, rights and liberties, material resources, knowledge, and self-respect, are necessary *whatever* one's goals happen to be. If Sally consistently values pain, disability, poverty, misery, ignorance, limited freedom, and humiliation, it is extremely difficult for most people to make sense of her beliefs and goals. Imagine, for example, that Sally told us she was buying a Harley-Davidson motorcycle *because* it would impoverish her, increase her risk for injury, cause her friends to regard her as irresponsible and insensitive, and generally make her life more difficult. What sense could we make of this? Sally may qualify as rational and yet consistently fail to *achieve* these primary goods most of us hold in common, but if she did not endorse or embrace them at all we would find it virtually impossible to understand not only Sally's goals but also her critical evaluation of anything. Thus, although Trappist monks embrace asceticism and a life of deprivation, they have as their ultimate values such things as spiritual wisdom, religious enrichment, and love for humanity. Theirs is not an outright rejection of all the goods mentioned, so much as an alternative appraisal of the means by which certain goods or ends are reached.

The procedural component of rationality involves adherence to certain logical rules of inference combined with the ability to formulate, revise, and pursue ends or goals in an intelligible manner. Integral for formulating and revising is the process of "deliberation," roughly speaking, the examination of one's beliefs, desires, habits, and values. Deliberation does not demand Cartesian asceticism, in which all unproven beliefs must be denied. Rather it involves a general tendency to excogitate, to consider the appropriateness of particular aspects of our lives. Which aspects are actually called into question will vary with circumstance, and clearly certain aspects will be less accessible because they lie deeper within our conceptual matrix. But without the capacity and the general tendency to deliberate, formulate, and revise our beliefs, desires, habits, and values, it is hard to know what it would mean to regard ourselves as rational.

Another part of this process of formulating and revising is the ability to recognize both evidence and inferences as compelling reasons for changing one's beliefs and behavior.[5] Though obviously there will be disputes over what should count as evidence or what beliefs and behaviors are entailed by a given inference,[6] differences in interpretation generally do not belie disagreement about canons for what constitutes rational thought. We can recognize Sally's ability to comprehend without *having* to agree with her conclusions.[7] Still, to qualify as rational Sally must be capable of critically examining the connections and relationships between various ideas, plans of action, and values and moreover be able to revise her ends or goals on the basis of her evaluation.

Of course, that Sally can carry out such a critical evaluation with regard to certain concerns—for example, getting dressed or her beliefs about pain—does not necessarily qualify her as rational. For these may be but isolated competencies, not indicative of the larger constellation of competencies that make rationality a global designation and that are necessary for comprehending, critically evaluating, and addressing the larger sweep of concerns that make up human existence. Sally might have severe rheumatoid arthritis and also be mentally retarded. Thus her capacities to discriminate between different kinds of pain and understand how various sorts of clothes affect her and her condition may make her competent with regard to those particular concerns, but not others. Of course, not all one's capacities come into play in every situation. What is needed to comprehend, critically evaluate, and decide what should be done will vary depending on the circumstances. A middle-aged teacher who hurts her back in the middle of the school day will need to work through a very different set of concerns than will an eighty-five-year-old widower whose back injury threatens his ability to continue living alone. Moreover, depending on one's reading of the situation and how various capacities reinforce one another, what *makes* for competence (in terms of qualifying as rational) may both take different forms and be configured with different capacities. That is, because particular capacities often interlace and support one another it is difficult to identify precisely which capacities must be present in any given situation to "produce" competence. It is in part this indeterminacy that makes it problematic, and in certain ways a misnomer, to speak of "the capacity for rationality" except in the most general ways. The reality, however, is that we do set a minimum threshold for the designation "rational."[8] For we understand that a general (albeit complex) constellation of capacities and competencies is sufficient for comprehending, analyzing, and making decisions regarding the wide range of concerns that arise within human experience.[9]

What then is the relation of all this to the capacity for autonomy? Can we say that if Sally enjoys continuity of self, accepts an intersubjectively accepted set of goods, and has met some threshold for procedural rationality then she possesses the capacity for autonomy? I think the answer is yes. In the first place, it is not clear what other general characteristics might be necessary to enable someone to reflect upon and endorse decisions in a way that expresses the kind of independent critical evaluation that characterizes autonomous decision-making. Perhaps, since *discerning* a person's capacity for autonomy often involves some form of inquiry, we might add to our list the ability to provide reasons for one's decisions and actions. But such an ability does not constitute a substantive amendment—even should it prove crucial for *defending* one's autonomous status. From a political standpoint the minimalist conception I have proposed has appeal because at the same time that it acknowledges the importance of nonarbitrary qualifications it recognizes the need for an inclusive rather than an exclusive threshold. Such a need arises because of the extreme importance attached to being regarded as the kind of being capable of making autonomous decisions. And so, just as the importance of not being considered "dead" leads us to a minimalist conception of "being alive," the fact that "having the capacity for autonomy" is what makes it possible to regard someone as a moral equal leads us to conceive of the capacity for autonomy as inclusively as is reasonable.

To take a step back for a moment, the question is, What does it mean to be autonomous? So far I have discussed the general qualifications that comprise the capacity for autonomy. What now follows is a discussion of conditions that can reduce or defeat a person's autonomous nature. Despite the natural tendency to focus on particular decisions and actions, I will argue that there are deep problems with local, synchronic determinations of autonomy.

Particular Aspects

Colloquially, we refer to Sally as living autonomously if we believe she is the ultimate judge of how she lives her life. We do not mean that she is unbound by any constraints or uninfluenced by her environment, but rather that somehow or other she is in control of her person as a whole as well as of her individual decisions and actions. That said, it can be quite difficult to distinguish between a nonautonomous Sally and an autonomous Sally who simply is making a nonautonomous (or *less* autonomous) decision. This is because conditions that reduce or defeat one's autonomous nature may do so to varying degrees. Moreover, a particular condition sometimes may compromise autonomy only in isolated instances while at other times abrogate autonomy for extended periods of time. Given this variability, a condition's effects on autonomy must be understood relative to particular circumstances. To paraphrase Joel Feinberg, even a very weak push can have the effect of a hurricane wind if one is unprepared for it and already off-balance.[10]

One difficulty with framing autonomy in this context-sensitive way is that it might be thought to imply that for an act or decision to qualify as autonomous it must be undertaken calmly and deliberately, in "a cool moment." But clearly this is not so. Sometimes our most deeply held beliefs, habits, and values are most truly represented in spontaneous and emotional behavior.[11] The assumption that the standard for autonomous decision-making should entail philosophical reflection and cautious deliberation reveals intellectuals' bias. If we see anger, fear, or improvisation as impugning autonomy we thereby deny the autonomous nature of many great and characteristic human accomplishments, whose absence would impoverish the scope and significance of autonomous action. We need only look to love or literature or art or experimentation more generally to see how often "a cool moment" fails to describe the process of autonomous behavior. Conversely, some of the paradigm cases of nonautonomous behavior are carefully and deliberately undertaken.

What autonomous behavior does demand, as part of rationality, is that Sally be able to recognize reasons for and against behaving in a particular way and be able to engage in behavior on the basis of her judgments. For without the ability to discriminate between good and bad, compelling and noncompelling reasons or incentives for doing X, and without the ability to act according to her judgments (assuming that she is free to do so), it is unclear how Sally can be thought of as self-governing.[12] This demand ushers in a discussion of the conditions that compromise the capacity for autonomy, rendering one either unable to recognize relevant incentives *or* incapable of acting in accordance with one's beliefs about them. A laundry list of such conditions might include fear, anxiety, exhaustion, neurotic compulsion, overwhelming desire, depression, delusion, insanity, anomie, diminished psychic continuity, and intoxication.

By definition, insanity and compulsion always abrogate the capacity for autonomy. As for the other conditions, they too may undermine the capacity for autonomy altogether; alternatively they may produce a more local loss of the capacity for autonomy or simply diminish one's capacity for autonomy but yet leave one above the threshold.[13] To the extent that conditions like anxiety, intoxication, and delusion give rise to particular incapacities,[14] they can impair the capacity for autonomy in a number of ways— just as vision may be impaired due to brain damage, retinal scarring, cataracts, or nerve damage.[15] Such impairments may be temporary, as with most narcotic intoxication, or more enduring, as with neurotic compulsion or clinical insanity. How these various conditions bear on the *exercise* of autonomy will be discussed in the next section. For now, though, the point is that how a particular condition will affect a person's capacity for autonomy varies greatly.

Take fear, for example. The effects that a given fear has on Sally's capacity for autonomy will depend on such variables as the specifics of the situation, her values, and her preferences. We can well imagine certain kinds of fear that would so paralyze Sally that she would be robbed of the capacity for autonomy entirely. Other fears might abrogate Sally's capacity for autonomy only with regard to particular areas of her life.[16] And still other fears may just "rattle" her so that while she would still be able to carry out critical evaluations she would be well below her normal level of functioning. Clearly, the various effects that fear, intoxication, and depression have on a person's capacity for autonomy are the sorts of things that must be determined empirically, and as such will be not only difficult but subject to normative (and oftentimes rather subjective) considerations.[17] Still, I think we can say generally that a particular condition *compromises* Sally's capacity for autonomy when it impairs her ability to carry out a critical evaluation and that it *undermines* her capacity for autonomy entirely when it robs her of the ability to formulate, revise, and pursue her ends or goals intelligibly or it so alters her state of consciousness that she ceases to be (sufficiently) connected to her established self.

Though I believe this to be a defensible position, it is open to two particularly strong challenges. The first challenge calls into question the appropriateness of conceiving of the capacity for autonomy as a threshold. The argument goes that if the reason we regard Sally as having the capacity for autonomy is that she can carry out a sufficiently critical evaluation and engage in behavior on the basis of her decision(s), then it is not clear why it should matter whether Sally is above some (normatively established) threshold. Either she is competent to carry out a critical evaluation with regard to the matter at hand or she is not. This is not to say that Sally must possess a *specific* set of capacities, only that she must meet the accepted level of functioning for any given issue. The more complex the decision, presumably the higher the level of functioning necessary to constitute having the capacity for autonomy. For example, Sally might possess the capacity for autonomy with respect to delegating a durable power of attorney, but not with respect to making actual decisions about medical treatment.

There are at least four general responses to this challenge. On the most basic level, it is simply impractical to reject a threshold standard for the capacity for autonomy. The sheer number and variety of specific determinations—classifying decisions according to their level of complexity as well as measuring a person's various capacities for autonomy—would prove unworkable. Second, such an approach essentially begs the political question how such determinations should be made and by whom. Anyone who has attended a committee meeting understands the infeasibility of a wholesale democratic process. And yet, given the bias and vast power imbalances within society, one runs an unspeakable risk in privileging some more select group to decide which decisions are sufficiently complex that they stand beyond the capacities of this or that group of people.[18] Relatedly, it is not clear who or what could legitimate the privileged status of that select group to begin with. Third, such specific determinations of capacity are problematic from a developmental standpoint, for often there is no clear distinction between an unexercised capacity, an undeveloped capacity, and the absence of capacity. How capacities are acquired and which ones are actually present is not clear-cut, and we should be wary of rigid designations— if only because of what we might suppress.[19] Fourth, the sorts of capacities necessary to critically evaluate disparate situations overlap tremendously. Though perhaps not generally acknowledged, the sorts of cognitive skills needed to critically evaluate personal relationships or make decisions regarding child-rearing are very similar to, and certainly no less sophisticated than, what is needed for arguably complex technical decisions. In fact the distinction between "intellectual activities" and "nonintellectual activities" is in many cases a false one. This is not to say that every person has the knowledge and experience and insight needed to make a good decision in every situation. But part of what is built into the notion of a normative threshold for the capacity for autonomy is that those who meet that level of functioning possess the critical skills necessary for understanding their own deficiencies and for making decisions that might be affected by those deficiencies. As I have suggested, part of what it means to regard Sally as a moral equal is to regard her as the kind of being who possesses such a threshold capacity.

A second and more sweeping challenge raises the question of whether autonomy is itself a viable concept. Take, for example, Jon Elster's discussion of adaptive preference formation with its metaphor of the fox and the sour grapes.[20] Adaptive preference formation refers to the adaptation a person's preferences undergo due to her perceptions regarding what is and is not attainable. In the strongest of ways, adaptive preference formation calls into question the possibility of autonomy by implying that social and psychological factors conspire to manipulate our judgment.[21] This impugns the very notion of self-governance by reducing it to the self-direction one could exercise in emerging from a thorny thicket, where one's path is virtually dictated by the conformations of the thicket. The possibility of autonomy is similarly challenged by critical theorists who charge that human behavior is an overdetermined product of an ideologically constructed self. On this reading, the influence of language, unconsciously acquired habits, and indoctrination with unreflected-on values early in life constitute the primary governing factors of a person's life and are the more powerful for their slow and uneventful nature. Because both values and rationality are seen as inseparable from ideology, the notion of genuine self-government loses virtually all meaning. There are, of course, less extreme critiques, ranging from charges of ideological hegemony to manufactured consent. The overall effect, however, is to severely challenge the presumption that most, or even some, individuals are capable of living autonomously.

I must admit that I do not quite understand how to entertain such critiques, whether they be forms of determinism or quasi-structuralism. For, in essence, these critiques ask whether we can meaningfully retain the concept of autonomy or believe that it has any real scope. Clearly this is not an illogical challenge, but it does call to mind George Burns's response when asked how it felt to be ninety-four years old: "Well, consider the alternative." The alternative here is to reject the belief that most individuals are autonomous and to assume that what now passes as self-governance is but a melange of conditioned and spontaneous responses. It is to render the notion of self-critical reflection meaningless. It is to deny that our choosings reflect anything more than happenstance reactions (however complex) to the decisions we face. Without the belief that self-government is possible what would be the point of deliberation?[22] In fact, it is not clear what deliberation would mean. It is also not clear what it would mean to speak of restoring a person's mental balance without it devolving into a political power play. On what grounds, for example, could we differentiate truly psychotic behavior from that which is simply *different* from our own? Moreover, without some notion of an autonomous self it is difficult to understand how we can reasonably tie moral value or significance to a person's actions. In what way are they hers beyond their simple physical connection?[23] We take people's ideas and values and decisions seriously in large part because we believe they were autonomously generated.[24] And so while it is perhaps conceivable to regard everyone (oneself included) as nonautonomous, to do so would demand a wholesale restructuring of not only the sorts of distinctions we draw between people and amongst decisions and ideas but also the way we attach meaning to the decisions and values and preferences of people. For how we understand ourselves and others is heavily influenced by our assumptions regarding the presence or absence of the capacity for autonomy and the extent to which autonomy is reflected in people's decisions and values and preferences.

We can, should, and do distinguish between, on the one hand, being a victim of ideological overdetermination and, on the other hand, simply being the product of influences. We understand that those with the capacity for autonomy can avoid being merely propelled by surrounding forces. An ideological victim suffers from nonauthenticity, substantially diminished power, and utter lack of awareness, whereas, by and large, the rest of us do not. One finds this distinction in legal statutes and theories of developmental psychology as well as in our interpretation of everyday social intercourse. We make a distinction between those who have the capacity to direct their lives and those who suffer from its absence. Exactly where one draws the line along the spectrum of levels of aptitude will vary among different schools of thought, as well as between individuals, but that a distinction exists is not a matter for dispute.

Of course it is rare for the previous challenge to be made with genuine equanimity. Seldom do those who see fit to challenge the existence of autonomy similarly question their own capacity for autonomy. Certainly within the medical environment the norm is for HCPs to place themselves beyond the fray when challenging the possibility of autonomous decision-making, somehow believing that their own intense professional socialization as well as the various pressures they are subject to do not affect *their* ability to make autonomous decisions. What makes this more than just an incidental observation is that the effect of such one-sided challenges is to deny patients equal respect. For the challenge to the authenticity of patients' decisions and values is not based on some procedural difference between how patients arrive at conclusions and how HCPs do. Rather it is based on their status as "patients"—often accompanied by differences in race, socioeconomic background, age, gender, and culture. The point is that one cannot treat a patient as a moral equal without according her equal respect, and challenging a patient's capacity for autonomy simply by virtue of her *patient* status can in no way be seen as equal respect.

Obviously, I have carried the discussion of autonomy only so far. I have not, for example, examined what makes a decision autonomous or argued that most decisions should be regarded as autonomous. I have yet to explain what characterizes a PSR matter, much less defended the importance of according autonomous patients final say with regard to PSR decisions. As these various issues are raised I hope to make it clear that important implications follow from the positions we take on these matters. For whether we see certain health care decisions as PSR and as "belonging" to patients will make an enormous difference in how HCPs are expected to behave and in how society should (re)structure the practice of medicine.

④ Kinds of Autonomy

It is common practice in health care to use a patient's past decisions (or behavior, more generally) as the *standard* for whether a decision is autonomous. Take the case of Alan, the HIV-positive patient described earlier. Alan's physicians challenged the autonomy of his decision to forgo certain procedures because, they pointed out, Alan had previously sought treatment. In addition to the mistaken assumption that seeking treatment is an all or none proposition, judging the autonomy of a decision by prior decisions is suspect on at least two counts. First, prior decisions, themselves, may not have been autonomous.[1] Second, it is often precisely when we have the opportunity to reflect upon, reassess, and restructure our value schemes that we change our minds; as such it is entirely consistent with autonomous decision-making to break from even long-established habits. This is not to say that we should not regard uncharacteristic decisions or behavior as red flags, alerting us to look deeper, to Alan's mind-set, to determine whether his behavior was autonomous. But by regarding past behavior as an indicator rather than a standard, we can be suspicious of radical changes while yet recognizing that the autonomy of a decision is a procedural matter. The question that remains is what procedural components characterize a decision as autonomous.

According to David Richards, my decisions and behavior are autonomous to the extent that they are the products of reflection and self-criticism. For this I must possess and exercise standards of self-critical evaluation that have been determined "not by the will of others but by arguments and evidence that [I have myself] rationally examined and assented to."[2] Clearly this does not require that I be able to conjure my ideas, values, and goals out of nowhere. Rather what it means is that I must entertain and act on desires and plans that I have self-critically evaluated. This allows us to conceive of my (autonomous) decisions and life plans as arising from my desires, but not *bound* to my immediate present desires.

Unfortunately, this description leaves much untold. For example, what is the exact relation between desires, rational deliberation, and autonomy? Living autonomously certainly does not require incessant conscious reflective analysis. But what is necessary? Lawrence Haworth argues that "normal autonomy" involves a critical competence that goes far enough in finding reasons for one's preferences without going to heroic lengths of deliberation.[3] Still this does not provide a very clear explanation of what (autonomous) deliberation involves, what sorts of reasons are acceptable, or what constitutes a sufficient degree of deliberation and how often it need be exercised.

Different schools of thought attempt to provide a procedural account for autonomous decision-making. Virtually all endorse some form of critical reflection as necessary for achieving autonomy, but there is a startling amount of diversity over the degree to which rationality, per se, is emphasized.[4] As mentioned earlier, the role of rationality is not unproblematic, for among other things it is not clear exactly how rationality can be a precondition for autonomous decision-making and yet avoid running roughshod over such decision-making. This dilemma is presumably part of what led Kant to define autonomy in terms of adherence to universal moral law. Contemporary writers' efforts to explain the deliberation process attempt to avoid Kant's retreat to an extracorporeal obedience of rational law. Some emphasize integration of desires, others authorship, and still others identification.

A particularly influential explanation of autonomous decision-making, the Dworkin/Frankfurt model, emphasizes *identification* using the language of higher order desires (HODs) and lower order desires (LODs). LODs "have as their object actual actions of the agent: a desire to *do* X or Y," while HODs "have as their object other LODs: a desire to desire to do X or Y."[5] If Sally's LODs included the desire to have a Coke or go to graduate school or listen to blues, her corresponding HODs (which are the products of higher order critical reflection) would be *to desire to desire to have a Coke, to desire to desire to go to graduate school, and to desire to desire to listen to blues.* On this model, Sally's decisions are autonomous insofar as her HODs endorse her LODs, and this process of identification is "not alien" to Sally. The question that this model leaves unanswered is what makes the process of higher order critical reflection "not alien"? That is, how can we tell whether the HOD that endorses the LOD is itself authentic, such that the *identification* is constitutive of autonomous decision-making? What is this mysterious process of procedurally independent indentification? John Christman refers to this as "the problem of incompleteness" and explains that what is needed is an account of what makes for an illegitimate external influence; that is, what would impugn the autonomy of the process by which HODs are formed?[6]

Christman's first proposal is that we employ a calculus of causation, whereby as observers we would decide how much weight an external influence should have on a person's higher order reflection. Christman's example of a calculus of causation that demonstrates diminished autonomy involves a dying woman who refuses treatment out of financial concerns raised by her son. According to Christman's calculus, the influence of the son's financial concerns constitutes an illegitimate influence. But presuming that the woman is competent, why should we think that her son's comments were either untoward or diminish the autonomy of her HOD? Economics are, after all, as much a part of reality as is pain or the quality of life. This seems to me a perfect example of how controversial any calculus of causation must be and how problematic it is to assume that outside observers can decide how much weight an external experience *should* have. Christman's rejoinder is that we employ such a calculus all the time. But do we do so correctly, and how often do our calculations involve something so significant as autonomy? That Christman ultimately admits that what qualifies as an illegitimate external influence may well rest on deep intuitions points to the inadequacy of using a calculus of causation to discern autonomous decision-making. For in the absence of general agreement regarding deep intuitions, it is at least dangerous to base the distinction between autonomous and nonautonomous decision-making on something that can be neither examined nor defended and is entirely external to the person whose decision-making is being judged.

Alternative proposals for characterizing illegitimate external influences are similarly not without difficulty. Take a second suggestion by Christman that an external influence is illegitimate if the agent whose HODs it influenced would not accept the role played by it and would be moved to revise the desire so affected were she to be made aware of that factor's presence and influence. An example of this might be the stress and pain a pregnant woman experiences during labor. Supposing that she would not accept the role played by stress and pain in her decision-making, stress and pain would count as illegitimate external influences that diminished the autonomy of her decisions. Aside from such practical concerns as how to identify all the factors that influence a decision or how to measure them, this proposal has other problems. The first is that ignorance or lack of insight might defeat the underlying thesis. For if Sally cannot or will not recognize that X influenced her, then she cannot or will not be able to admit the reduction of her autonomy. Identifying an illegitimate external influence relies upon Sally being able and willing to revise her desire. The problem is that in many instances this is not the case. People deny the significance of influences all the time; take, for example, the marketing of pharmaceuticals. Physicians roundly declare that because they have been "trained in science" they are able to see through and ignore the ploys of drug representatives who ply them with free lunches and gifts. It is clear, however, that if freebies were ineffective at influencing the "scientific choices" of physicians pharmaceutical companies would have stopped them long ago. Social relations and emotional ties are even subtler, and hence more problematic. Add to this the additional layer of internal autonomy-limiting influences (e.g., extreme compulsiveness or highly ingrained habits) and it becomes increasingly clear that the attempt to explain autonomy via "identification with one's desires" leaves us essentially where we began: *What is the nature of the process that gives rise to autonomous decisions or desires?*

A second and more telling problem concerns the assumption that HODs de jure subordinate LODs in the authentication process that determines autonomy. One form of this objection, developed by Bernard Berofsky,[7] stresses that endorsement must be conceived in terms of a three-dimensional appreciation of the psyche. Among other things, this means not underemphasizing the significance of our first-order natures,[8] or ignoring that the "intellect" sometimes serves as little more than a handmaiden for rationalizing transient, albeit powerful, passions.[9] So, if we believe that autonomy describes that which is our true nature, we should be careful not to artificially limit or oversimplify what constitutes that nature.

A position that sidesteps some of these difficulties is that of Gerald Dworkin, who holds that what is critical for autonomy is "the capacity to raise the question of whether I will identify with or reject the reasons for which I now act."[10] This position addresses autonomy as a global rather than a local concept and thus avoids having to characterize particular decisions as autonomous or nonautonomous. It seems to me that an important implication of this view is that once we are satisfied that Sally is above the threshold capacity for autonomy, there is no subsequent process for inquiring into the autonomy of her decisions except to question whether the conditions (internal or external) surrounding Sally's decisions have conspired to undermine her capacity to be autonomous.[11] What makes such a conclusion so extreme (and unattractive for some) is that to challenge that capacity one must show more than simply that Sally did not appear to exercise certain capacities, more than that she was "unduly" influenced by a particular factor, more than that she disregarded her more lasting interests. One must show that Sally was lacking the capacity to, in Dworkin's language, "raise the question of whether I will identify with or reject the reasons for which I now act." Otherwise, the most we can say is that by *our* standards she is acting unreasonably. To challenge Sally's autonomy further we must call into question her capacity to carry out the higher order reflection that is involved in creating procedurally independent conclusions.[12]

It seems to me that something like this is right, that once we have assured ourselves that Sally has satisfied our conditions for having the capacity for autonomy there is no further avenue for challenging the autonomous nature of her decisions. So, in Alan's case, unless we can show that his fear of having a lumbar puncture *undermines* his capacity for autonomy about this decision, we must accept that his decision is an autonomous one. This shifting of the burden of proof can be defended on at least three grounds.

First, and at the root of the issue, is the basic inaccessibility of the decision-making process. Even those of us who pride ourselves on our reflectiveness and ability to rationally evaluate issues often find ourselves at a loss to explain how we made a given decision. Exactly how did we choose *that particular* name for our child or our pet? Yes, we have reasons. But why did those reasons predominate over others that presumably would have been equally defensible? It is not any different with more important decisions, either, like how we *really* made that tough decision about the right thing to do. When it comes right down to it how, *really,* did we choose between competing responsibilities? How do we *really* decide what counts as a good or better reason? It seems to me that how a person comes to make a decision is sufficiently mysterious that we should be cautious of arrogant presumptions that we can qualitatively distinguish the various influences that generate a decision, much less an autonomous decision.

Second, a model for autonomy that resists dissecting individual decisions has appeal because there is much more to human existence and expression than can be accounted for by rules of reason and acceptability. In the same way that great literature sometimes ignores rules of grammar and syntax and yet communicates brilliantly—perhaps in a way that would not have been possible had the rules been adhered to—so, too, does the fullness of human action require a flexibility with regard to "autonomous action."[13] That some people will regard Sally's behavior as extreme may be of little consequence to its place in the larger scheme of human activity, wherein expressing the humanness we value may take many forms.[14] There is nothing so rigid and narrow as to believe that a certain value scheme, or an appreciation of benefits and costs, is "right" to the exclusion of other appraisals. True, we must employ some normative considerations to have standards at all, but this normative requirement can occur at some remove, namely, when we say that Sally has the capacity for autonomy. Of course the more important, the more risky, the more irreversible a decision, the more we will want to scrutinize Sally's mental state. For we will want to be clear that great and preventable damage is not suffered unwittingly. But the vagaries of human expressiveness and creativity make external calculations of decision-making intractably problematic.

A third and related matter involves the political aspects of external calculations of decision-making. Attempts to define a person's authentic as opposed to alien interests are fraught with mixed intentions. The standards used for "autonomous decision-making" often prove inseparable from the values and goals of those carrying out the calculation. In fact it is hard to avoid the conclusion that attempts to define people's "authentic" interests and desires often have to do more with imposing or promoting certain values and asserting power than they do with discerning "authenticity."[15] It is in part this tendency that makes paternalism so suspect and that ought to give us all pause should we see someone coming down the road to do us good. This is not to deny that some paternalistic interventions will have positive consequences for the recipient, but the moral and political statement being made sets an unjustified and dangerous precedent. The message is unequivocal: We who would intervene do not believe that your decisions should be taken seriously . . . at least not until they conform with ours. But without *clear proof* that a decision is nonautonomous this is no more than power politics.

Now perhaps Sally does qualify as having the capacity for autonomy and simply is not exercising that capacity.[16] But often there is no clear process for discerning this and no way to safeguard any proposed process from the unconscionable and predictable abuse that would result. Even the most cursory look at how the tradition of medical paternalism has played out for women, people of color, the elderly, and the poor confirms such apprehensions. By demanding that would-be paternalists disprove a patient's *capacity* for autonomy, we shift and strengthen the burden of proof for denying people equal respect, for denying their status as moral equals. It is not only that decision-making is mysterious and paternalistic interventions suspect. The importance of protecting patients' status as moral equals until the basis for that status is refuted is crucial from a moral standpoint. But also, how can we expect people to take responsibility for their lives if we do not treat them as beings who can be trusted to make their own decisions?

Before we go on to explore autonomy as a capacity, consider the following case as an illustration of the difficulties inherent in assessing the autonomy of decision-making. Imagine trying to figure the calculus of causation or determine whose vantage point should be privileged for carrying out the calculations. Also note how dialogue is used to examine and respect the exercise of autonomy.

Dialogue 2: A Labor of Love and Respect

At thirty-seven years of age, Amy has been a nurse-midwife in a quiet midwestern community (population fifty thousand) for about ten years. Amy likes to have at least one meeting with prospective mothers and members of their support systems during the first trimester. It is also her policy, whenever possible, to meet with them regularly throughout pregnancy for both medical and emotional support. Amy uses these visits to monitor the women's development and provide them with information about pregnancy as well as labor and delivery. Amy also works during these encounters to establish a professional and personal relationship with each patient. Additionally, Amy helps mothers design an individualized birth plan and encourages them to take responsibility in preparing themselves for the birth of their child.

Amy is careful to ensure that all high-risk pregnancies are managed in coordination with an obstetrician, and of course she abides by the state law requiring midwives to have a licensed physician as back-up to assume responsibility if the situation requires it. Amy is known for encouraging her patients to be informed and prepared for the various events surrounding pregnancy and childbirth. Amy is also known for being supportive of natural childbirth and for encouraging involvement of members of the woman's support system throughout the entire pregnancy and birth process.

Up until August 15 Amy had had a relatively uneventful five-month relationship with Jack and Juanita Ewing, both of whom were twenty-eight years old and in good health. Jack and Juanita taught at the local high school and this was their first pregnancy in their five years of marriage. In discussing the various options, Jack and Juanita told Amy they wanted to have a "natural childbirth" at the local hospital birth center—located at the far end of the obstetrics and gynecology ward. In particular they wanted to have a vaginal birth and to avoid both episiotomy and pain medication if at all possible. On Friday evening, two days before Juanita's due date, Amy got a call from Juanita to say that she had begun to have irregular contractions every ten-fifteen minutes and that this had been going on for the past few hours. The two of them spent about twenty minutes on the phone reviewing the standard events in early labor, the danger signs Juanita should watch out for, and the importance of hydration, good nutrition, and rest. They also went over again the couple's birth plan. Then next morning was the fifteenth. About 10:00 A.M. Jack called to say that Juanita was having contractions every ten minutes, that she was feeling them low down, and that Juanita said it felt like "the real thing." When Amy arrived at the birth center about 11:00, Jack and Juanita were already in one of the birthing rooms, excited and a little nervous.

AMY: Heya! How ya feelin'?

JUANITA: Real good so far. I was so excited last night. But I did catch a little sleep between contractions. Me and Jack had a light breakfast this morning like we talked about, and then went for a walk. I guess that must've done it, 'cause by the time we got back the contractions were coming closer together—and that's when Jack called. Luckily, we had time last night to go rent *Fried Green Tomatoes* in case labor went on for a while today. I hope you like that movie. We brought all sorts of food too—fruit, Popsicles, yogurt, bagels, brownies, you name it, I think we have it. I always get so hungry when I get excited. It's alright to eat, isn't it?

AMY: Sure. It's important to stay well-nourished. But you don't want to fill yourself up. The key thing is to stay comfortable and relaxed. Remember, the more at ease you are, the easier it'll be for your body to do what it needs to do. And yes, that's one of my *favorite* movies. How about you, Jack? (*then, with a bit of irony and a smile*) Everything "under control"?

JACK: Yup! We got just about everything we need: food, movie, video camera, music, books, pregnant woman in labor. I see clean sheets on the bed. I think the only thing we need is boiling water and we're set.

AMY: OK. Just let me listen to you and the baby, Juanita, check your cervix, and then I'll leave the two of you alone for a while.

(*Amy does a quick physical exam as Jack looks on.*)

AMY: Everything looks good. I'd say you're at about three centimeters right now. We just have to wait and let nature do its thing. I'll plan on checking in on you now and again just to make sure you're comfortable. I'm gonna go call your physician to let her know where we are. If you need me I'll be just down the hall in my office catching up on some paperwork. If I can clean off my desk in time maybe I'll even watch some of the movie with you. I really love that part where she goes and gets the honey.

(*By 5:00 that afternoon Juanita is pretty uncomfortable. Her contractions are roughly five minutes apart, and she winces and squeezes Jack's hand with each spasm. Amy is in the room along with Erik, one of the birth assistants. A doptone machine for monitoring fetal distress, an IV, and various other pieces of accessory equipment are set up just in case they are needed. Jack and Juanita's physician is on call at the hospital and will be there until midnight. Up to this point everything has gone smoothly, though both Jack and Juanita are getting rather anxious, and the experience of being in labor is a little more "out of control" than Jack would have liked it to be.)*

JUANITA: How much longer do you think this is . . . whew! . . . gonna be?

AMY: It's just so variable. I've seen babies pop right out and I've seen others that have really needed some coaxing. The main thing is to try to relax as best you can and remember that this is a process. So many people in medicine think of labor as something simply to get *through.* Instead of focusing on outcome, try to concentrate on the process, on the meaning this has for you, the specialness of labor as an experience *all by itself.* (*Juanita nods.*) Anyway, you're doing all the right things. Just keep it up. When I checked a few minutes ago you were at five centimeters. Those last five centimeters might take an hour, or four or five, or, you never know, it might go on all night. The thing to remember is that all of us are going to be here with you, helping you through this.

JACK: Honey, do you want to take a warm bath? They say that helps.

JUANITA: Maybe later. Could you rub my back, though? . . . a little further down. Oh, that's nice—maybe just a little harder. Ahhhh.

AMY: If you're at all thirsty, you might think about having some juice— maybe even eating a little something. It's important to keep your strength up, and sometimes it'll even take your mind off the discomfort.

JUANITA: That would be good. There's some cranberry juice in the little fridge right there and some yogurt would be nice right now. My sister, Elizabeth, made some special black walnut, fudge, and peanut butter brownies for me, "for when I get hungry during labor," she said. But I think I'll pass on them. (*making a face at Jack*) What was she thinking?!

ERIK: (*motioning Jack to stay with Juanita*) That's alright, Jack, I'll get it. Amy, Jack, do you want some too?

JACK: No, I'm fine. Thanks.

AMY: Yes, please! Now that I think about it, I never had lunch. Between all that paperwork and the movie, I forgot to eat. How unlike me.

(*Five more long, uncomfortable hours have passed. It's 10:00 and Amy, Erik, and Jack are all still in the room with Juanita. Juanita's sister, Elizabeth, has driven in from the southern part of the state and has been there since about 8:00. Despite a long bath, lots of back rubs, and even a short nap, Juanita is in a great deal of discomfort. Juanita is sitting up on the bed, propped up by three pillows.*)

JUANITA: How much? (*pant*) How much is it now? . . . Ugh!

AMY: It's about six, maybe six and a half. You're getting real close.

JUANITA: (*sobbing a little*) I'm in so much pain . . . mmh!! . . . How much longer will it take? I don't think I can . . . I don't think I can do this much longer. It hurts!!!

AMY: I know. I know it hurts . . . you're doin' real good, though.

JUANITA: I need something. I need something for pain.

JACK: Honey, remember we agreed that you wanted to have the baby without any medication.

JUANITA: Jack, it *hurts!!* (*Now she is crying.*)

JACK: It's alright. It's gonna be alright.

ELIZABETH: Jack's right, Juanita. I thought I was gonna die when I had my first baby. But here I am. You'll be OK. (*sympathetically*) It's *supposed* to hurt.

AMY: (*gently*) Remember what we talked about, Juanita. Try to keep your breathing steady. Don't let the contractions consume you. Think of each contraction as a wave, and let's just get to the top. You know it's gonna come down. You know it'll ease. Use the time between the contractions to rest. (*soothingly and softly*) Breathe, and try to relax.

(*This works for about half an hour. Then Juanita has a forceful contraction that makes her body go almost rigid with pain.*)

JUANITA: Agh!!! Oh Jack! Jaaaaaack!!

JACK: (*looking very anxious and not sure what to do*) I'm here. I'm right here.

JUANITA: (*really crying now*) It hurts so bad! Agh!! There it goes again. Jack, I can't take this, I . . . agh!!!

AMY: Juanita? Juanita, you need to try to listen to me now. We're all here, and we're here to help you through this. I know the contractions are bad. But between the contractions where does it hurt?

JUANITA: (*sobbing*) It's worst in my back, and it shoots . . . oh! . . . it shoots down the back of my legs.

AMY: OK. That's why we're here. Try laying on your side. Jack, can you massage her legs while Elizabeth and I rub her back? I know it's hard, Juanita. But we're all going to help you, and then you're gonna have a beautiful baby.

ERIK: (*softly*) Juanita, would you like some juice to sip on? And I can put some quiet music on if you'd like.

JUANITA: Please. That would be nice. Mmh! You're all being so good . . . ugh! . . . I'm sorry, it just hurts so very much.

JACK: That's OK.

AMY: Remember? This is what we've talked about, what we've been preparing for. This is good pain. It's going to bring your baby. You're giving birth to a whole new person. You're entitled to hurt. Just remember that this is all part of the process, the same process that brought you into the world some twenty-eight years ago.

JUANITA: (*panting hard*) I just don't know if I can do it. Oh . . . it hurts so much!

AMY: I know. Let's just take it one contraction at a time and try and make it work. You and Jack have come a long way on this and I know how hard you've worked to keep yourself healthy and have the kind of birth you wanted. We just have to keep working a little longer. How's your back? Are your legs starting to feel more relaxed?

JUANITA: A little, but it still hurts. Ow Oh-Ow!!

AMY: If you can't take it one contraction at a time, take it one *breath* at a time.

(*Amy and Jack together try to help Juanita get into a breathing pattern, to help move her focus off the pain. Juanita works at this for a few minutes, but then is jarred by a strong contraction. Juanita is now screaming almost at the top of her lungs.*)

JUANITA: Agh! Aaagh!! Make it stop!!! Make it stop!!!

AMY: Try to visualize something peaceful, something other than the pain, Juanita. I know it's hard. Jack, maybe if you sat behind Juanita and held her, that might help. I want to feel how dilated the cervix is.

(*As Amy checks Juanita's cervix her contractions ease. But she continues to be in a lot of pain.*)

JACK: Amy, can't we give her something for the pain? She's really in a lot of pain. Maybe just one epidural. Whatever you think's appropriate. But she needs *something!*

AMY: (*gently, as if she were smoothing Juanita's hair*) You're almost there. Your cervix is just under seven centimeters. We're on the back stretch now. You're doing real well. Let's just keep working through each contraction.

JUANITA: (*exhausted and crying out*) It hurts!! They're coming so fast! It hurts!! Jack! Do something!!

JACK: (*somewhat frantic*) Amy, what should I do?!

AMY: (*gently and calmly*) Jack, why don't you go ahead and get off the bed. Juanita? Sometimes it helps to change positions. Maybe try getting on your hands and knees. And remember, just keep trying to find a focus other than the pain. Elizabeth, see if you can help Juanita . . . maybe if you helped her to the bathroom. Sometimes sitting on the toilet for a few contractions or taking a shower helps. The more relaxed we can help Juanita to be, the easier and less painful the birth is going to be. Erik, why don't you help Elizabeth and Juanita. Jack, while they're in the bathroom can I talk with you for a minute?

(*Amy wants to discuss some things with Jack, but she also wants to give Jack a breather, as he seems to be getting really nervous. Amy and Jack move to the corner of the room and Amy pours them each some juice. They talk quietly.*)

JACK: (*imploringly*) Juanita *needs* some pain medication!

AMY: Let's see how she does for a few minutes and then let's talk about it. I know this is difficult, but . . .

JACK: You heard her! She can't take this anymore. I *know* Juanita. She doesn't like pain. You can't let her go on like this. It's not right.

AMY: Jack, remember, we talked about this. About how it's normal for women to have this much pain and that most women can make it through without needing medication. What we have to do is help Juanita *through* the pain.

JACK: But she doesn't want to *be* in pain!

AMY: Jack, I know it's very hard for you to see Juanita in so much pain. But you have to remember that this is part of the natural experience you both wanted. We talked this out. You saw films and read about what it would be like. Juanita understood that it would be hard and that she would need our support to make it all the way through. And that's just what she needs now, Jack, *our support*. She needs you to help her. This is the kind of experience she wanted.

JACK: This is what she thought she wanted . . . what we thought we wanted. But it's so much harder than I ever thought it would be.

AMY: Look at her now, Jack. (*They both look across the room toward the open door of the bathroom where Juanita is seated on the toilet.*) She's breathing. She's more relaxed. She can do it. She is doing it. Lots of women, lots of couples, have a hard time sometime during labor. It's natural for you to feel the way you do. You love Juanita and you don't want to see her hurt. But you have to ask yourself what all this means, and will mean, to the two of you. I think what Juanita needs is reassurance. (*Amy pauses, giving Jack a moment to think about what she's said.*) Often, pain has as much to do with fear as it does with actual physiological sensation. We can help her *through* the pain, even the really intense pain. And by doing so, the two of you can have the kind of birth you've worked for for so long.

JACK: That's easy for you to say. It's not *your* wife. It's not *your* body that's in pain. Pain's different for everyone. You don't know what she's going through. I don't know if I *want* a natural experience anymore. I just know I want Juanita and the baby to be healthy, and that includes Juanita not having to be in the kind of pain she's in right now.

AMY: Jack, Jack, calm down a little. I really do know this is difficult for both of you. And I want to say right up front that I'm not going to keep pain medication from Juanita if that's what the two of you decide she wants. Right over there on the counter I have some Vistaril, which is an anti-anxiety medicine. We have a syringe with Nubain all set up if she needs an injection of narcotics to ease the pain. *And* I've got everything we need to give Juanita an epidural if the pain gets so bad that it needs to be blocked entirely. There's a nurse-anesthetist just down the hall. But part of my job is to help be your advocate, and sometimes that means pushing you to put things into a broader perspective. If all that childbirth was about was losing twelve pounds and walking away with a healthy baby, it wouldn't be anything more than a medical procedure. But it means something more than that. I'm not at all trying to make Juanita suffer. I'm just trying to help her have the kind of childbirth that the two of you wanted.

JACK: (*frustrated*) Look, I don't know what I want. I just don't want Juanita to be in any more pain. We picked you to help us not just because we needed someone to deliver the baby, but because we thought you would help us do what we wanted.

AMY: This is a hard time. But it's going to be over soon. The two of you can make it through this. And my experience tells me that if you can carry through with the kind of birth you wanted to have, you're both going to be really pleased.

JACK: What are you saying, that we can't change our minds? We can't come to our senses and realize that this is more than we bargained for?

AMY: I'm not saying that at all. But *isn't* this what you bargained for? Isn't it the case that you wanted to experience, really experience, having a child, in all its intensity? I'm not saying that if Juanita gets pain medication it'll be a less valuable experience. But it will be different from what you had hoped. There's no doubt this is a hard thing to go through. Just try to be patient. You're doing really well.

JACK: I don't know if I can. But anyway it's Juanita, not me, that matters. She's the one who has to go through the pain. She should be the one to decide what to do, what's best for her. We need to ask her what *she* wants.

AMY: We can ask her, and I think we should. After all, it is her decision. But remember, this is a hard time for Juanita. She may decide things now in the heat of the moment that she'll later regret. And I'm not saying that she shouldn't make the decision, but that we should help her as much as we can so that she doesn't have to make a decision that both of you might come to wish she hadn't made. It's important to give her real options. (*Out of the corner of her eye Amy sees Juanita stepping out of the shower.*) There, she's just about to come out of the bathroom now. Why don't you go talk to her, and I'll come over in a few minutes. If the two of you decide that she wants pain medication, then that's what we'll do. But do think about it. Oh, and when you go over, would you ask Erik to come over here? Thanks.

(*After Jack goes to be with Juanita, Erik walks over to Amy. Shortly thereafter, Amy and Erik are joined by Elizabeth.*)

ERIK: Really? I thought she had decided beforehand that she didn't want any pain medication.

AMY: (*tilting her head to the side*) Well, that was then and this is now.

ELIZABETH: Do you think my sister's in any condition to be making that kind of decision? It's not that I want to see her in pain. But my sister is one stubborn person and I had the impression that she had her heart set on a totally natural childbirth. I mean, you know all about women and labor way better than I do. But for months whenever we talked on the phone about it, Juanita would go on and on about how she was going to experience the whole thing, start to finish, au naturel.

ERIK: I've only been with you for a few births, Amy. And you're in charge. But if you give her pain medications . . . Look, it may turn out just fine, but you might catch a lot of flack and maybe even a lawsuit for violating her autonomy or something like that. (*Erik raises his eyebrows and then continues half-flippantly, but also half-seriously.*) A couple of the obstetricians I work with say that once women are in labor all bets are off . . . and you have to admit (*Erik looks over toward Juanita*), that's not exactly the textbook picture of an autonomous decision-maker.

ELIZABETH: Oh, I'm sure Juanita wouldn't do anything like that. She's said such good things about you. I'm just concerned that it wouldn't be what she wanted.

AMY: Well, in my experience this is the most difficult part of labor, and if she can get through the next hour or so I think she's going to be OK. But to be honest, I'm not as sure as either of you that a woman's being in painful labor *means* that her decisions are any less autonomous. I'm not sure I could tell you what being autonomous is exactly, but I'm not at all convinced that simply being in labor is enough to undermine someone's capacity to *be* autonomous. I'm not saying that Juanita over there on the bed is exactly the same as the Juanita from yesterday. But humans are pretty complex beings. And it seems to me that if we want to know whether Juanita as she is right now is capable of making an autonomous decision about whether or not to have pain medication, then the only way to find out is by talking to her. We need to find out where she's at. I think you're both right that Juanita did feel very strongly about having a natural birth. But unless we're really convinced that Juanita's present decisions are actually nonautonomous, it seems to me that we have to abide by the decisions she makes *now*—with the understanding that she may well regret those decisions at a later point in time. But let's see what she says first.

(*Amy and Elizabeth walk over and kneel on the floor so they're pretty much at eye level with Juanita, who's lying on her side as Jack, laying alongside her, cradles her swollen belly with one hand and her head with the other.*)

AMY: (*very gently*) So how ya doin' there, Mom?

JUANITA: (*breathless and with a helpless look in her eyes*) OK, I guess. The contractions slowed a bit. But my back still hurts and I feel a lot of pressure in my vagina.

AMY: Would you like some wet towels on your forehead? How does it feel when I put some counterpressure on your back? . . . better?

JUANITA: (*moaning*) Ugh, a little . . . is there anything I can get to ease the pain?

AMY: There is. In fact we've been discussing that just now. The question is whether pain medication is something you really want right now. In the past when we've talked, and I gather—from what your sister's said—when you've talked with Elizabeth, too, you felt very strongly about having a "natural birth" without any medication. None of us want you to have more pain than you have to, but you need to decide whether you really want pain medication or not, whether you feel you really need it. Sometimes it has more to do with fear than it does with pain.

JUANITA: (*tensing with her eyes shut*) What do you think?

AMY: (*gently but matter-of-factly*) I think it's your decision. But I also think that you can do this, that you can have the kind of birth you wanted—*without pain medications*. Your body knows how to deal with this. It's opening up and stretching as we talk. What you've been experiencing so far is entirely normal. Lots of women feel just like you do. And I know it's scary for you 'cause you don't know what's coming next or how long it'll last. But you're really doing well, you and Jack both. The good thing is that this is the shortest part of labor. I know it hurts and that you're feeling afraid to push. But believe me, you're going to be able to push right through the burning. And once you get to that stage it'll be over before you know it. I do have pain medications just over there on the counter. They're all ready to go. (*Amy pauses, but neither Juanita nor Jack says anything. Amy then continues.*) If you're thinking that you're going to want some Nubain, which is a narcotic, then we should give you an injection right now. And we can give you just half a dose and see if that helps. Are you with me here, Juanita?

JUANITA: (*her eyes still shut*) Uh-huh.

AMY: I've also got an epidural injection set up and all ready to go—I just have to call for the nurse-anesthetist. But that would mean starting an IV *right now,* and you'd have to wear a blood pressure cuff, too. We've talked about all this before. So you know there are some risks associated with anesthesia. I have no reason to think that you would have any complications. But it's important for you to remember that they *can* happen. (*Amy pauses and looks to Jack, who arches his eyebrows as if to say that this whole thing is beyond him. Amy continues.*) You and Jack, more than anyone else in this room, know what you want and what you need. I'm here, and so are your sister and Erik, to help you have your baby the way you want to. If pain medication is what you want, then that's what we'll do. But in that case we should start the process now. You're not yet at eight centimeters and it's a good time since you're a bit more at rest. (*Amy waits a moment to see if Juanita wants to say anything. She doesn't and Amy continues.*) *But* . . . if you still want to do it without any pain medication, all of us are here to help. We'll give you massages. We'll breathe with you. (*jokingly*) We can even get out your sister's brownies. (*Juanita smiles through her pain and opens her eyes to look at Jack.*) What's important for you to know is that you're not alone here. Whatever you decide is OK. But you do have to make a decision.

JUANITA: What do *you* think, Jack?

JACK: I don't know. I've never done this before. We both wanted to do natural childbirth, but . . . but it's hard to see you in so much pain. I'll agree with whatever you decide. (*Juanita looks at Jack a little skeptically.*) Really! How do *you* feel right now?

JUANITA: Better, I guess. But that's because I haven't had a major contraction in about five minutes, just a bunch of small ones that are so close together it's almost like one big long unending contraction. (*Juanita pauses to catch her breath and as she does so she winces a bit.*) We *are* really close, I guess. Maybe if I walked around a bit we could speed this baby up, hey? (*Juanita laughs tiredly. She then looks to her sister, who smiles and reaches out to smooth Juanita's hair. Juanita then looks back to Jack before finally turning to Amy.*) Whew . . . OK. I guess I'm ready to give it a try. (*smiling*) I don't think I'm really up for any of Elizabeth's brownies. But maybe some juice. (*Her hair matted with sweat, Juanita lifts an arm toward Jack.*) Jack, help me up, would you?

ELIZABETH: I knew you could do this, sis.

JACK: (*gently, but anxiously*) Now, honey. If it gets really bad and you can't take it anymore, you'll let us know, right?!

JUANITA: (*smiling exhaustedly*) Uh-huh. I'll probably scream a lot, anyway. But you'll know when I can't take it anymore.

AMY: (*gently*) Yeah. We'll know.

(*About forty-five minutes later, at 11:34, Juanita gave birth—without pain medication—to a healthy seven pound, eight ounce boy whom they named Joram, after Juanita's great-grandfather.*)

Autonomy as Capacity

Part of what makes the preceding case so challenging is that the clinical criteria for gauging Juanita's capacity for autonomy are far from clear-cut. But even if we could identify such clinical criteria, and were right to understand being autonomous as rooted in the capacity to carry out a rational and procedurally independent critical evaluation (along with having continuity of self and accepting an intersubjectively accepted set of goods), there remains the question of whether we can really characterize most patients as autonomous. Before answering, we should be careful to avoid identifying the procedural aspects of rationality and hence the capacity to be autonomous with the habits of twentieth-century intellectuals.[17] For not only is it unclear that intellectualism is the appropriate model for autonomy, the very procedural independence of intellectuals' habits of deliberation is far from proven. As Jacques Ellul writes, intellectuals "absorb the largest amount of secondhand, unverifiable information; they feel a compelling need to have an opinion on every important question of our time, and thus easily succumb to opinions offered them by propaganda on all such indigestible pieces of information; they consider themselves capable of 'judging for themselves.' They literally need propaganda."[18] Obviously, the point is not to indict intellectual reflection, but rather to question the assumption that the intellectual class is an appropriate paradigm for autonomous behavior.

This said, what *are* the trappings of having the capacity for procedurally independent decision-making, and do most adults possess them? Clearly, substantive independence is not necessary; it is no sign of incapacity that we choose to do what others do. Nor is it a necessary component that we act consciously, for unconscious habits may manifest autonomous behavior just as artfully as conscious deliberation. We often make customary that which we most fully endorse. Just as one need not examine the lyrics of a familiar song each time one chooses to sing it, one need not reexamine every option when making a familiar decision. This is not to deny that many habits and values are adopted nonautonomously. We acquire values and habits long before we can even articulate them, much less examine them critically. But as we mature, we *do* acquire that ability to critically examine our lives, to reflect on our habits, values, and our belief systems. In fact, part of maturing is learning that our decisions are open to critical reflection and that we are capable of performing that examination. This is not to say that we do exercise our capacity for autonomy as fully as we might. At any given moment much goes unquestioned, just as some people never question certain beliefs. But most of us do possess and exercise the capacity to act autonomously. We weigh options, make (cognitively) highly sophisticated judgments about friendships, work, and current events, and perhaps more importantly just generally are prone to reassess our decisions once a problem or conflict is perceived.

The difficulty, of course, lies in establishing that such decision-making is indeed autonomous. For there is much that we adopt nonautonomously. Otto Neurath provided an apt metaphor for how we reexamine and reconstruct parts of our lives without having to be in intellectual dry dock. The idea is that a boat can be rebuilt while still at sea, so long as one does it but a few boards at a time. The one drawback with this metaphor is that it assumes an independent shipwright whose designs for rebuilding stand apart from the ship itself, and in the present context we are at pains to identify that independent engineer in ourselves. In other words, because most planks of our intellectual ship are nonautonomously acquired, to defend the rebuilding process as "autonomous" we need to show whence comes the autonomous critical perspective that carries out the reexamination. How can I stand apart from everything else that makes me *me* so that I can reconstruct *me* in a way that is procedurally independent from all the things that make me *me*?[19] How do the issues even get raised to consciousness?[20] My guess is that answers to these questions bring us as close to mysticism as any issue we are liable to encounter with regard to autonomy.

It seems to me that Dewey was on the right track in arguing that consciousness has its roots in "conflict," arising as an attempt to resolve disharmony between impulses, one's environment, and established habits.[21] We become aware of some personal or social issue or the back of our knee when the previously existing relation of forces becomes unharmonious, no longer unified. Consciousness then allows for deliberation, a process whose goal is effective reintegration of the various interacting forces. If we understand consciousness in this way, then by combining conscious reflection with (1) a facility to entertain alternative possibilities, (2) the ability to make reasoned calculations based on the strength of one's values, beliefs, and priority schemes, and (3) the capacity for procedural independence outlined above, perhaps we arrive at a general explanation of how consciousness and autonomous examination occur. Clearly the origins of this capacity remain obscure. But one need only look to love, aging, art, even humor to recognize that the capacity for autonomy is not alone in this regard.

The question is whether such an understanding of autonomy describes most adult patients. What common experience tells us is that it does, that most adults can consider alternative possibilities, make reasoned calculations, and arrive at decisions in a procedurally independent manner. That such capacities are not always exercised does not thereby call into question their existence. In fact, to do so would challenge many basic social conventions, from the legitimacy of legal and moral responsibility to the value we place on democracy. The moral and psychological distinctions we make between children and adults is based on more than just judgment; centrally at issue is the capacity for autonomous behavior that children lack (in varying degrees) and that most adults possess. This distinction holds equally for "intellectuals" and "nonintellectuals" and is independent of social or professional status. No doubt, certain people are more prone to exercise their capacity for autonomous behavior, just as various circumstances are more likely to evoke such behavior. But empirically, I think it is borne out that the vast majority of adults do indeed possess the capacities at issue.

What I will turn to next is the claim that a class of decisions should be seen as PSR and that what it means (in part) to respect a person's autonomy as a moral equal is to respect her prerogative to make PSR decisions.

Primarily Self-Regarding Matters

If the exercise of a person's autonomy is to be respected then PSR decisions must be defended first, for they help define a person's boundaries and identify her as an autonomous individual. As decisions that "belong" to the individual, PSR decisions differ from mere legal arrangements and contracts that guarantee the right to make certain decisions. PSR decisions constitute a minimum sphere of dominion, without which the very concept of self-government fails. This is not to say that others cannot or should not try to influence Sally's PSR decisions, decisions such as whether to refuse medical treatment, endanger herself, or limit her opportunities. But unless at the end of the day Sally (alone) has final say, she can hardly be thought of as self-governing.

For some, of course, it is question-begging to call certain matters or decisions PSR. The *relational argument*, as I will call it, claims that because individuals, no matter how isolated, do not exist apart from society it is implausible to distinguish matters that are PSR from those that affect others. To be sure, relationists do not deny that certain actions are more or less other-regarding. Rather, the relational claim is that, despite case-by-case variation, no decision either stands separate from its consequences or can be viewed uniformly as more self-regarding than others. Even with rather private decisions that do not trespass the rights of others—such as how to care for oneself, how to spend one's money, whether to become intoxicated—relationists balk at the classification "self-regarding." In particular, they object to the common reliance on rights to properly locate decision-making. They claim that the very language of rights is unduly atomistic, that it fails to take into account the context and narrative that give situations and decisions their meaning. According to the relational argument the scope and breadth of interactions (amongst both people and actions) make it impractical if not impossible to relegate certain decisions to a private self-regarding realm. For relationists, the intricacies and intimacies of our social interrelationships are such that no decision, and in fact no person, can be isolated from the rest of society.

This general critique can take any number of forms. One approach is to argue that a self that is not defined by its ends, commitments, and relationships to others is essentially unrecognizable.[22] With this reasoning, such a radically detached self is not only implausible but it also renders genuinely communitarian enterprises impossible. A related criticism targets the atomistic foundation of so-called "primacy of rights theories"[23] for their tendency to ascribe rights unconditionally without recognizing a similar unconditional principle of belonging or obligation. This line of argument suggests that because society is necessary for human development, we cannot at once value the essential properties that define human beings as bearers of certain rights without also valuing those relations and conditions that are necessary for developing those properties.[24]

An even broader critique of the traditional philosophical model of the individual argues that it is incoherent to base universalized principles on disembedded and disembodied notions of autonomous selves. Discussions about rights and contracts must be contextualized, it is claimed, and the historical failure to do so—that is, to be concerned with the details of relationships and narratives—has led to "a privatization of women's experience and to the exclusion of its consideration from a moral point of view."[25] More concretely, this tradition of using a decontextualized model of the individual for universalizing theories has relegated properties such as caring, education, health, and emotions to a private realm not subject to public safeguards.

The relational critique can be extended to a still larger frame of reference if one understands the very notion of rationality in terms of one's community.[26] With this reasoning, because communities are the basis for shared understanding, rationality itself is a product of the norms we embrace and relationships we form. To the extent that we want to develop rationality we must then dedicate ourselves to the practical task of fostering the solidarity, participation, and mutual recognition that forms the basis for a genuine community. The more of our relationships we can accommodate, the more potential we have for realizing an ever greater sense of community and the more powerful a sense of rationality we embrace.

Clearly, the issues raised by these relational arguments are wide-ranging and cannot be dealt with in a few paragraphs. Many philosophical traditions have struggled and continue to struggle with the relation between the individual and the community, as well as with the overall framework for interpreting rationality and justice. What I can do is suggest ways we might understand the conception of autonomy I have developed thus far, so that it is not thought to either ignore or trivialize the relevance and importance of these relational concerns, and then explain how PSR decisions can be reconciled with the relational argument.

To begin, there is no question but that the function and value of autonomy are embedded, intrinsically and pervasively, in the context of relationships. Autonomy's value derives from its place within the matrix of our conception of what it is to be an interacting, responsible, principled, responsive human being.[27] To my knowledge there is nothing in my characterization of autonomy that suggests otherwise. Nonetheless, I think relationists are mistaken to suppose that relationships that involve a sense of caring, belonging, personal emotional obligation, and so on *have* to exist for autonomy to develop, much less be sustained. Without question, most autonomous beings, and often those we value most, embrace and exemplify these relationships. But is the relation here contingent or necessary? It is not at all clear that the sorts of conditions necessary for autonomy to develop—

as opposed to certain virtues to develop—require the full range of relationships that relationists claim. If relationists are right, then valuing and respecting autonomy *does* logically entail valuing and respecting the relationships they claim give rise to and sustain autonomy. In this discussion, however, I have argued that to qualify as autonomous, all Sally need do is exhibit continuity of self, accept a minimal intersubjectively accepted set of goods, and possess a threshold capacity for procedural rationality (and all that that entails) with regard to how to live her life. But if this conception is correct, rarely will the broad spectrum of relationships argued for by relationists be *necessary* for developing, exemplifying, and ensuring the existence of autonomy. And if they are not necessary, then valuing and respecting autonomy does not create an obligation to embrace and protect all such relationships. Essentially, this argument is driven by the empirical judgment that most individuals could achieve autonomous status in the absence of relationships generally thought of as caring, expressing personal emotional obligation, and so on.

Relationists might reply that relationships that involve caring and belonging simply are constituent of an autonomous existence, that is, of our lives and values as they really exist, and as such should not be discounted merely because they are contingent. We should understand their contextual role and appreciate that relationships (and the obligations they entail) give autonomy its importance by creating the context in which autonomy functions. There is no doubt that this assertion has intuitive appeal, but at base it turns on a misunderstanding of what autonomy is about and what it represents. Autonomy's value has to do with its being a necessary condition for many of our most important values as well as assumptions about people. And this is true independent of any particular social relationship. This is not to say that we should reject outright the central role ascribed to social relationships by various authors. Relationships do frame and contribute to autonomy's role within society, and thus to its prominence. They help explain the respect and protection we wish to accord individuals within society by providing the context in which autonomy is viewed. Any conception of autonomy must recognize this, and in that sense be broad enough to "cover" those aspects of relationships foundational for human autonomous existence. Thus, various relationships (child, friend, community member) must be taken as given for there to be a context for Sally's autonomy to develop and operate. We are undeniably all intimately connected. Our actions affect each other in significant and far-reaching ways, even when they are the result of our most intimate and personal decisions— decisions that many of us would want to characterize as "ours to make."

Hence the question is not whether interconnections exist, but who should decide (under normal circumstances) what force these interconnections have (or should have) in our decision-making.

Clearly many decisions are community decisions, just as sensitive negotiation can avert controversy in many situations.[28] But can we really accept that no decisions "belong" to the individual?[29] If no decision can *ever* count as PSR, then all questions of dominion will be left to some social/legal process. The effect of this, however, is to deny individuals any moral claim to particular decisions and to place any possible distinction between the personal and the political on dangerously shifting sand. For by forfeiting the notion of PSR one concedes that no decision whatsoever deserves protection from the prevailing political winds. Obviously, what counts as a PSR decision must rely at some level on a deep intuition about what the individual, and no one else, has the prerogative to decide, for few unequivocal criteria demarcate PSR boundaries. But this is not an indictment of the concept of PSR so much as a signpost to its roots in our conception of an autonomous individual. Would you surrender *your* claim to decide how you will treat your own body or to decide how much significance various interconnections have (or should have) in *your* personal life? Chances are your answer will be "no." But why? Not simply because of some instrumental calculation of utility. As a rule physicians may well make better medical decisions than patients, just as extended families may make better matchmaking decisions than spouses-to-be. Rather, our answer relies on our understanding of what it means to be treated as an autonomous being, as one who is capable of making life decisions and determining the meaning that the ramifications of her decisions and actions have and should have.

Does this mean that with regard to PSR decisions respect for autonomy precludes valuing the sorts of relationships that situate autonomy? Certainly not. Many relationships deserve to be respected and promoted both in their own right and in the interest of fostering autonomy.[30] Nor is there anything hard-hearted about what it means to be autonomous. Nothing prevents an autonomous person from being (more) virtuous, and surely nothing suggests that one is more autonomous for being more selfish or uncaring. Nonetheless, in terms of autonomy it is irrelevant whether one acts so as to benefit other people, and in terms of PSR matters respect for another's autonomous decision should not depend on the kindness or virtuousness of that decision. What it is to regard Sally as "the author of her own projects, as engaged in living her life in a way that has creative significance and value to her as her own" is to recognize that *she* will decide whether to act meanly or with affection, in a prejudicial fashion or with equal consideration for others.[31] This is not to deny that certain relationships entail special obligations; nor is it to say that we should not esteem Sally for being considerate of others. One hopes that Sally will be aware of the far-reaching consequences of her actions and that she will take them into consideration when she deliberates and makes decisions. That is all for the good. But being nice or helpful or considerate is not part of what makes Sally autonomous, nor should these traits be accorded special status under the aegis of valuing and respecting autonomy. Now, it may be that higher levels of autonomy entail more comprehensive reexamination, revision, and consistency with regard to one's guiding principles, and in that case it is conceivable that more autonomous individuals have a tendency to be more virtuous. But even this is a tenuous assumption in that it supposes the complexity of an individual may be brought under consistent control by the advanced development and exercise of autonomy. At any rate, autonomy does not have value or importance because it conduces to beneficence or virtue.

Consider the following case as an illustration of not only what is meant by a PSR decision but also how an HCP might go about investigating a person's capacity for autonomy and respecting her PSR decisions. Note how by entering into dialogue Richard's doctor develops their relationship in a way that increases the meaning of their interaction, thereby making it possible to genuinely respect Richard's autonomous decision.

Dialogue 3: Having Final Say

Richard Bitone is seventy-four years old and has been in the Veterans Administration hospital (VA) for approximately six months. He was originally admitted for chronic renal failure to the VA's long-term care facility, but two months ago he had a heart attack, or myocardial infarction (MI), that was life-threatening. After a brief stay in the intensive care unit (ICU), Richard was placed on the general medicine ward, where he remained until four days ago, Monday, December 17, when he was transported back to the ICU with his second MI in two months. Because their home is 150 miles away in Thomasboro and Richard's wife, Betty, is an elder at their local church and active in civic affairs, Betty is able to make the drive to visit her husband on only Tuesdays and Fridays. On those days, Betty spends six or seven hours with Richard and also speaks with the VA staff who provide Richard's care. It has become clear to the staff that when Betty is around, Richard very much defers to her. Consequently, the directives that Betty has helped to set in place for Richard's care are heavily influenced by Betty's values.

Like many VAs around the country, the hospital where Richard is being treated is a teaching institution for various surgical, psychiatric, and internal medicine residents. Dr. Stacie Fuller is just finishing her first two-month rotation at the VA. Stacie is a first-year internal medicine resident (also called an intern) who is on call this weekend. As of Monday, Stacie will return to the local private-pay hospital to work for the next four months and will not return to the VA until early summer. Stacie is one of the more conscientious and warm-hearted interns, and it has been Richard's good fortune to have been under her care since his first admission to the ICU in October. As both Richard and Stacie are aware, the VA, like many hospitals, for all intents and purposes shuts down on weekends. By 5:30 P.M. on Fridays, the VA is a very quiet place. For the few harried residents and the skeleton staff of nurses who run the VA on weekends, the primary goal is simply to keep anything from going horribly wrong before 8:00 Monday morning.

It is now 7:30 on Friday evening and the VA is especially quiet since it is just a few days before Christmas. As usual, Richard's wife has spent the day talking with Richard, as well as getting beaten by him at both cards and Scrabble. Betty has been gone now for about an hour and is on her way to spend the weekend with relatives, some five hours away, so that she can spend all of Christmas day with Richard. Since Richard's admission to the ICU four days ago his condition has remained stable, but there is no doubt that his most recent MI has significantly weakened his heart and further compromised his cardiac output. Stacie is finishing her rounds on the thirteen patients for whom she is responsible before retiring to the doctors' lounge to order some Chinese food and relax a bit. Stacie is hoping to finish Alice Walker's *Temple of My Familiar,* which she started to read just before coming to the VA in October. As Stacie stops to talk with Richard, he comments that Walker is one of his wife's favorite authors.

RICHARD: Betty once showed me an essay that woman wrote on the civil rights movement that I thought was pretty good. But . . . I don't know. I think most of that stuff is for women, if you know what I mean. Like that Cary Grant movie my wife likes so much . . . what's it called? . . . *An Affair to Remember,* but deeper than that.

STACIE: I never saw that. But I've been a fan of Alice Walker's for a long time, being a "womanist" and all. (*Richard looks confused; but rather than explain what a "womanist" is, Stacie shifts topics.*) So anyway, did you have a nice time with your wife today?

RICHARD: Oh yeah! I beat her four games of gin in a row. And in Scrabble I got a triple-word score for *Xerox.*

STACIE: You must make some good money winning all those games.

RICHARD: Oh no! My wife's a religious woman. She doesn't believe in gambling—calls it the Devil's business . . . no, we don't never bet. (*laughing*) But I beat her just the same.

STACIE: Well, I guess that's a good thing.

RICHARD: You a religious woman, doctor?

STACIE: Well . . . not really. I was raised up in a church. Used to go every Sunday. And I loved to sing in the choir. But . . . well, by the time I was sixteen or so . . . I still liked the people, but . . . I don't know . . . I just didn't seem to fit anymore. They were always proud of me and all. But I always felt that somewhere deep down they expected me to take a backseat to men. (*Stacie looks down at her white doctor's coat, back at Richard, and then smiles.*) And as you can see for yourself, I tend to be a little more willful than that.

RICHARD: (*smiling back*) Well, you helping me alright.

STACIE: (*Stacie gives Richard a little nod.*) I appreciate your saying that.

RICHARD: Me, I'm not that much of a religious person. Used to be, me and Betty would really get into it, her wantin' me to go to church; me wantin' to go fishin'. I always figured that when I'm done workin' my time belongs to me. The thing is that Betty just has a lot more use for prayin' than I do. I just sort of accept things as they are, figure I do my best, and what happens just happens.

STACIE: My grampa was sort of like that. He used to say that seeing so much death during the war made him realize how little control you really had over your life.

RICHARD: Yeah. I understand that. When it's time to go, the good Lord will come and take ya. Ain't no use puttin' up a struggle. Like they say, the dealer's always got the upper hand. (*Richard pauses, as if deep in thought, then looks up at Stacie intently.*) Do you believe that, being a doctor and all?

STACIE: (*thoughtfully, really pulled into the conversation now*) Depends what you mean, I guess. I've certainly seen people go who didn't *have* to. My grampa, he died at home, sleeping in *his* chair. His heart just quit one day, like it knew he was ready. But I also knew a guy in medical school who committed suicide, and I just can't believe it was his time yet. I think that sometimes people don't know any better and just give up when there's still time left on their meter. (*Stacie catches herself thinking about her grandfather and comparing his death to her classmate's. Then, realizing that this conversation may be about something that Richard needs to talk about, she quickly shifts the conversation back to Richard. A little more attentive now than before, Stacie studies Richard.*) Is there something particular that *you* had in mind?

RICHARD: Well . . . I guess since about Tuesday I've been doin' a lot of thinking. You know, I didn't fall out or anything when I had my heart attack on Monday. I just had these pains right here (*he points to his chest*) and I called the nurse and they rushed me down here and said I was havin' another heart attack. I wasn't really scared, but I thought that was it. But then you came down, just like that first time, and got me all squared away. Well anyway, when Betty came in the next day and I had to rest, she started talking about how she had spoken with Dr. Raphael, who recommended starting me on some kind of rehabilitation and new drugs and some other stuff. And I just got to thinkin' that I'm too old for this. My kidneys don't work that well, now my heart doesn't work right. I mean, I've still got my mind and all, but I'm starting to think that it's time to go and . . . that's alright. I've never been all that big on Christmas. I always did it up big for the kids. But I'd just as soon pass on it, ya know.

STACIE: It sounds like you've been thinking about this a lot. Have you talked with your wife about it?

RICHARD: No . . . I don't think she'd really . . . well, really listen. She'd think I just needed to rest and would feel better when Christmas came. So, I haven't really said anything.

STACIE: Hm. Is there anyone else for you to talk to?

RICHARD: Well, me and my son, Keith, are pretty close. But he and his wife are down in the Caribbean on vacation. It's their ten-year anniversary. He's a civil rights lawyer out in L.A. and he hardly gets any time off. They called on Wednesday when they heard I had another heart attack, but we couldn't really talk much long distance. And to be honest, since I hadn't really pulled my thoughts together yet, I don't even know what exactly I could have told him. They're not due back for another two weeks, but they said they'd try to call on Christmas so they could talk to both me and Betty. I guess you're really the only one I've told. Most people don't ask, don't really want to know.

STACIE: Yeah, I know. Well, what are you thinking of doing?

RICHARD: I think I'm wantin' to have one of those, whaddaya call 'em, "do not revive" things put on my chart—so when I get called, y'all just let me go.

STACIE: Are you really sure that's what you want?

RICHARD: I think so. (*Richard pauses, thinks for a minute, and then goes on.*) Thing's aren't really lookin' up, and I figure it's best not to go out like that Karen Ann Quinlan girl, all skin and bones, hooked up to machines, not doin' anybody any good, but no one willing to call it quits. I've had a good life. My Betty, she'll miss me, but she's younger 'n me and got lots of people back in Thomasboro. If there's ever a good time to go, I guess this is about as good as any. Ya gotta go sometime.

STACIE: Whewwww . . . that's a pretty big decision. Do you at least plan to *try* to talk to your wife about it? I mean, how do you think she'd feel?

RICHARD: Well, my wife and me are two real different people. She'd probably try to talk me out of it. And who knows, she might succeed. But it wouldn't be because that's what I want. Betty has this way of gettin' things done *her* way, and I'd just as soon have this one go my way.

STACIE: (*hesitantly, not wanting to offend*) Don't you think it would bother her when she found out? That you didn't talk to her about it?

RICHARD: I don't see why she has to find out. It's my decision, isn't it? I could just say that no one was to know.

STACIE: Well, it's not really that simple. In hospitals things get around. There are so many people involved in your care that it's virtually impossible that it wouldn't get back to her at some point. It . . . it *is* your decision, but it does involve other people. You just can't avoid that. (*troubled, but realizing that this isn't really her problem*) Um, well, who knows. Maybe this won't really be an issue. If you and Dr. Raphael can talk it out in the next week or so, maybe he can even help you work something out with your wife.

RICHARD: I thought maybe you could take care of this.

STACIE: I wish I could help. But this is my last weekend here at the VA. As of Monday I'm back at Mt. Zion, and I won't be here again until the summer.

RICHARD: I meant tonight. Can't you put it on my chart?

STACIE: You mean put a do not resuscitate order on your chart *tonight?!*

RICHARD: Um, yeah. That's what I had in mind. You're my doctor, aren't you?

STACIE: Uh, yeah. But I don't know if I . . . I've never done this before . . . and I'm just not sure that we should do it just like that.

RICHARD: Well, I've pretty much made up my mind, and it seems to me that whoever's supposed to do it just needs to do it, that's all.

STACIE: Whew . . . um . . . wow! Uh, I'm sort of caught off guard here. I really wasn't planning on this, uh . . . I'll tell you what . . . um, let me go make a phone call, and I'll be back in about half an hour. There's some things I need to find out.

RICHARD: Well, I won't go anywhere 'til you come back. But I would like to get this settled tonight. You never know what's gonna happen.

STACIE: (*walking away, she says quietly to herself*) You sure don't!

(*Stacie goes off to the doctors' lounge and calls her senior resident, Ralph, who is in another part of the hospital. Ralph explains that he's never had any direct experience initiating do not resuscitate orders and suggests that Stacie bring it up with the hospital ethics committee at their January meeting. Normally, the next person to contact in the chain of command would be the attending physician on call. This evening, however, the on-call physician is Dr. Tchula, with whom Stacie does not get along very well. So instead, Stacie calls Dr. Mark Pearlman, who is the chief attending physician for the internal medicine division of the VA. He is apparently out to dinner, so Stacie has him paged. While she waits for Dr. Pearlman to return her call, Stacie orders some carry-out from the Szechuan restaurant down the street, leaves some money for the food with the security guard at the door, and makes her way to the library. It is an hour before Dr. Pearlman returns her call. By this time Stacie is back in the doctors' lounge finishing her dinner as she reads through some articles and textbook entries on DNR. From the VA physician handbook, Stacie has already learned that the hospital policy is fairly straightforward. All that is required to initiate a DNR is evidence that a competent patient—or appropriate surrogate—has requested a DNR order and authorization of the order by an attending physician.*)

STACIE: Thanks for calling back. I'm sorry to bother you on a Friday night.

MARK: (*patiently but firmly*) That's alright, Stacie, what is it?

STACIE: (*somewhat nervously*) Well, Dr. Pearlman, one of my ICU patients, a Mr. Richard Bitone, wants me to put a DNR order on his chart *tonight*. The reason I'm calling is that I've never done this before and . . . um . . . well, the handbook says DNRs need to be authorized by an attending physician . . . and . . . um . . .

MARK: Well, is he competent?

STACIE: As far as I can tell.

MARK: Do you have any reason to think that he's not competent?

STACIE: Actually, Dr. Pearlman, no. I talked to him for about half an hour tonight and he seems as with it as you or me. I think you know him. He's the guy who came in about six months ago with renal failure, had an MI just after I started in October, and just had another MI this past Monday.

MARK: Oh yeah. Nice fellow, in his seventies, right? I've talked to his wife a few times.

STACIE: Uh-huh. Well anyway, he seems to have thought it out pretty well, but the thing is that he hasn't said anything to anyone else about it, not even his wife. She's off on a trip somewhere this weekend and not due back until Christmas—that's four days away. And his son's off in the Caribbean. I'm *particularly* worried since it sounds like his wife would object to him having a DNR order. This is his second MI in two months *and* since it was just four days ago that he had it, between now and Monday is when he's at the greatest risk for having a rupture of his ventricular wall. I mean, it is his decision, but . . .

MARK: Does it have to be done tonight?

STACIE: *I'd* rather it wasn't. But he's pretty insistent. I told him I'd get back to him half an hour ago. The thing is, he doesn't want his wife to even know about the DNR . . . I don't know what he expects. I told him that in a hospital like this it's virtually impossible for things like that not to get around and that one way or another his wife would find out eventually. But he still wants it done tonight. And I'm just worried that something's gonna happen to him between now and when she comes back on Tuesday.

MARK: Well . . . hospital policy is that so long as a patient is competent he has the right to request a DNR order at any time. Usually, it goes through his attending physician, and if there's a question about competency or something like that, sometimes the ethics committee will get involved. Who's his attending?

STACIE: Dr. Raphael.

MARK: I don't know when Dr. Raphael's in next. Monday and Tuesday are pretty much down days, it being Christmas and all. I'm on call tomorrow and Sunday and he's already asked me to cover for him over the weekend . . . he might not be in until after Christmas. This really isn't the best time to be dealing with this.

STACIE: Believe me, Dr. Pearlman, I know. This is my last weekend. As of Monday I'm back at Mt. Zion. The problem is that he really wants it done tonight. I looked at the hospital policy along with a bunch of articles from the library. As far as I can tell, unless there's serious reason to believe that the patient's mental functioning is impaired, either physiologically or psychologically, we have to honor his request as soon as he makes it. That's what the ethicists say, that's what the courts seem to say; it's even what the VA handbook says. (*Stacie pauses.*) To be honest, I really don't have any reason to think that Mr. Bitone is in any way impaired, but . . .

MARK: You said you've never done this before, right? Who's the senior psych resident on tonight?

STACIE: Kim Bodle, I think.

MARK: Well, why don't you give Kim a call and have her come do an evaluation. That way we're sure, and it'll be good for you to see how to handle this sort of thing in the future. Assuming Kim finds Mr. Bitone competent, you can initiate a DNR as of tonight and I'll come in tomorrow and authorize it. Does that sound OK?

STACIE: Yeah. Thanks . . . I would've asked Dr. Tchula—she's on call tonight—but I don't think she's the best person to be dealing with Mr. Bitone, if you know what I mean.

MARK: That's alright. I understand how these things go. Well, if you have any more problems, you can give me a call. I'm at home now and should be up 'til about 11:30. Otherwise, I'll see you sometime in the morning, OK?

STACIE: Thanks again, Dr. Pearlman. Good night.

(Stacie calls Kim and explains the situation. After a bit of resistance Kim agrees to talk to Mr. Bitone. Stacie walks back to the ICU.)

STACIE: Sorry I took so long. I had to talk to Dr. Pearlman and it took some time to get a hold of him. You still want to take care of this tonight, huh?

RICHARD: Yeah. I think so. You got the form for me to sign?

STACIE: Well, it's not quite that simple. Seeing that you haven't had a chance to talk this over with your wife or even Dr. Raphael, um . . . well . . . I just want to be sure that this is really what *you* want, and that you're ready to make this decision . . . mentally, I mean.

RICHARD: I thought I was pretty clear.

STACIE: What I mean is that . . . and there's no offense intended here . . . uh, I asked one of the other doctors here, Dr. Bodle, to come talk to you first. Dr. Bodle is a senior resident in psychiatry and has a lot of experience with people who when they're sick, or around the holidays, get depressed and . . . don't always make the best decisions for themselves.

RICHARD: Are you trying to tell me you think there's something wrong with my mind?

STACIE: Not at all. It's just that this is a very serious decision you're making, and since I'm the only one you've talked with about it, I just want to make sure that . . . well, that you're as . . . *clear* . . . as you seem to be. Kim's a very good psychiatrist, and basically she's just coming down to talk with you. In fact, that's her now.

(Kim strides into the ICU, and upon seeing Stacie smiles and gives a sort of half salute.)

KIM: Well, hello there stranger.

STACIE: Hi. Thanks, I really appreciate your coming over. (*turning to Rich-*

ard) Mr. Bitone, this is Dr. Kim Bodle, who I was just telling you about. Kim, this is Mr. Richard Bitone. I told Mr. Bitone that you were coming over to talk with him, but not because we thought he was crazy . . .

KIM: (*smiling and jokingly*) *I'll* be the judge of that.

(*Kim pulls up a chair and sits so that she is at eye level with Richard.*)

RICHARD: I don't know, this doctor looks pretty tough.

STACIE: Should I go and come back later?

KIM: No, that's fine. I'm sure Mr. Bitone, here, would just as soon have two women waiting on him rather than one. (*At this, both Richard and Stacie smile.*) So, Mr. Bitone . . . I need to ask you some standard questions and then we can just talk. Do you know where you are right now?

RICHARD: (*smiling and jousting back a little*) In the presence of two very attractive young women doctors, I'd say.

KIM: (*turning toward Stacie*) I like this man! (*turning back to Richard*) Now, Mr. Bitone . . . in addition to being in the presence of two attractive young women doctors, do you know what kind of institution you're in?

RICHARD: The VA hospital.

KIM: Do you know what the date is?

RICHARD: Let's see . . . today's Friday and Tuesday is Christmas . . . so that makes today the twenty-first, right?

KIM: That's right. Do you know who the president of the United States is?

RICHARD: Hillary Clinton, last I heard. (*Richard chuckles and Kim shakes her head.*)

KIM: Please repeat these three words after me: *chair, hippopotamus, rifle range.*

RICHARD: *Chair, hippopotamus, rifle range.* (*turning toward Stacie*) Mm, I don't know about this . . . where'd you get her?

KIM: Please count backward from 100 by sevens until I tell you to stop.

RICHARD: 100, 93, 86 . . . uh, 79, 72, um, 60—uh, 65 . . .

KIM: That's good. Now can you tell me why you're here at the VA?

RICHARD: Well, basically, it 'cause . . . ya see, I originally came in with kidney problems. Somethin' about protein and . . . uh, I don't know what. But then about two months ago I had a pretty major heart attack, and then I had another one about four or five days ago.

KIM: How old are you right now?

RICHARD: I'm seventy-four.

KIM: Mm, that's still pretty young. Can you tell me why it is you want to put a DNR order on your chart? You know, for a man your age there's still a lot that medicine, even surgery, can do for you.

RICHARD: Well, I guess it's like I was tellin' Dr. Fuller before. I just figure that the way things are going, I'm not gonna be getting much better. It's not that I *want* to die, but . . . well, I know how I don't want to live. And I don't want to spend years dyin' slowly while y'all hook up tubes to one part of my body after another. If I get better, that's just fine with me. But if I'm gonna go, I'd just as soon have the Lord take me quick. (*Richard arches his eyebrows and looks at Kim half-jokingly, but also half-suspiciously.*) Don't start gettin' any ideas. I'm not askin' anyone to try to kill me. I had enough of that in the service to last me a lifetime. But if I have another heart attack, then I think that's a sign that my time's done here, and I'd best move over and make room for someone else.

KIM: Dr. Fuller tells me you haven't talked with your wife about this.

RICHARD: Nah, it'd just trouble her if I did. Betty's not like that. She wants to fight everything 'til she gets her way. Me, I got more sense than that. (*Richard chuckles, but with a hint of sadness.*)

KIM: Don't you think it'd bother her if something happened and she found out?

RICHARD: Oh, she'd be upset for a while. But . . . she'd get over it. Wouldn't have much choice, would she?

KIM: What about your kids?

RICHARD: They'd understand alright. They're more like me than she is.

KIM: Hm. Mr. Bitone, do you think any of your decision has to do with your just having had this heart attack? Sometimes, major setbacks like that can be *very* disturbing, and yet in a couple of weeks, or maybe a month, you might feel real differently about it.

RICHARD: Mm, I don't think so. You gotta remember, I'm seventy-four years old. I've been around the world. I've played honky-tonk piano and raised children and been married for forty-six years. You're at the beginnin' of all that. I'm at the end. I don't have any regrets. It's not that I don't have anything to live for. It's just that . . . well, I believe that nature takes its course. And part of what you learn as you get older is how to know when you just gotta stand back and . . . well, let nature *take* its course. And that's how I feel now. You're young. It's different. You've got all these things you wanna do, and you're gonna fight 'til you get to do 'em. I've already done that. Doesn't that make sense to you?

KIM: Yeah, it does. The concern that I have, though, and that other people have, is that perhaps this decision isn't characteristic, or that it's somehow the product of depression. A lot of people get depressed around the holidays. And you *are* far from home. We do our best here, but it's not much of a supportive environment. I'm just worried that if we went ahead with this DNR order and something happened . . . well, that it didn't need to happen that way. Maybe we could've worked something out so that you felt more of a reason to fight a little longer. Or at least that if we waited until you'd had a chance to talk with your family about this . . . there'd be more of a consensus about your decision.

RICHARD: (*starting to get a little huffy*) I'll admit that I don't like Christmas much and it's not exactly home here. But I *am* a grown man, and I've got a pretty good idea about what's important and what isn't. With all due respect, it's not your business to be decidin' what's best for me. Once you get inside a hospital all of a sudden people think you can't decide things for yourself anymore. Why's that? *You tell me.*

KIM: Well, I'll admit that part of the reason I'm here is because you're in this bed. But you have to remember that people aren't used to being sick. For a lot of people going to the hospital is a pretty traumatic experience . . .

RICHARD: You think any more so than gettin' shot at or losing your job? Or gettin' married? If you'd had to deal with Betty's mother *that day,* you'd *know* what traumatic was!

KIM: You have a point. But it's different here.

RICHARD: As far as I can tell, the only thing that's different is that y'all have the power to keep me from makin' my own decisions. And that's not right.

KIM: Well, that's not what we're trying to do here. I'm not saying that there aren't doctors who do that. But we're just trying to make sure that you're in a sufficiently stable state of mind to make the kind of decision that's in your best interest. It's not that we're trying to make you do what we want you to do. But this is a pretty serious decision you're making, and it could upset a lot of people if we let you make it without being sure that you were competent and informed when you made it.

STACIE: Mr. Bitone, do you know exactly what a do not resuscitate order *means?*

RICHARD: As far as I know, it means that if my heart stops, y'all won't try to start it again.

STACIE: That's pretty much it, but you realize your heart could stop for any number of reasons. Some of them would only require a minimum of intervention to treat the underlying problem. We might just need to sort of give you a jump start, maybe an injection. If you signed a DNR order it would prevent us from even the smallest intervention. Is that really what you want?

KIM: Another thing you might think about, Mr. Bitone, is just postponing this decision at least until your wife comes back. I understand she's been very involved in helping arrange your treatment regimen.

RICHARD: Nah. I don't wanna do that. I want to get this done tonight. It seems to me that I should have the right to decide how I'm gonna live, and that includes what y'all do to me. Unless you're trying to make me out like I'm crazy or somethin', I don't see what right you have to keep me from making those decisions. I'm old enough to be your grandfather, both of you. Don't they teach you in medical school that you're supposed to respect your patients' wishes? Or don't they do that there?

KIM: I understand your frustration, Mr. Bitone. But that's what we're trying to do. It's sort of like checking someone's ID at the bank to make sure that they're the right person making the withdrawal. It may seem a little disrespectful at first. But when you think about it, aren't you sort of glad that they check everyone? You wouldn't want someone else taking money out of your account would you?

RICHARD: (*pointing to Stacie*) She's seen me every day since I had my first heart attack. That's two months. Are you sayin' she's not sure I am who I'm supposed to be?!

KIM: Not exactly. It's more that we just want to make sure you're protected, that all the money you've been saving is . . . well, that . . . uh . . . I guess we *are* trying to make sure you're who you're supposed to be. Because, with something as important as your life at stake, and us being responsible for your well-being, it's not something we want to make a mistake about.

RICHARD: (*now quite frustrated but recognizing that the power rests with Kim and Stacie*) So?! Am I who I'm supposed to be, or don't I get to make my own decisions anymore?!

KIM: (*somewhat apologetically*) I see no reason to think, Mr. Bitone, that you're not who you're supposed to be. I didn't mean to imply that you weren't. But it's my job to make sure. (*Kim stands up and smiles. Richard just watches her.*) Say, before I leave, can you tell me the three words again that I asked you to repeat a few minutes ago?

RICHARD: *Chair, hippopotamus,* and *rifle range.* (*then, impatiently*) Is that it?

KIM: That's it. Well, I wish you well, Mr. Bitone. (*Kim quietly reaches out and shakes Richard's hand.*) I hope everything works out like you want.

STACIE: I'll be back in just a minute, Mr. Bitone.

(*Stacie follows Kim out of the room. They talk quietly as they move down the hall out of earshot from Richard.*)

STACIE: So, whaddaya think?

KIM: I think he reminds me of *my* grandfather, too—stubborn, knows what he wants. I'll tell you, Stacie, I can see why you like him so much and want to protect him from making a bad decision. But he's as with it as you or me, at least as far as I can tell. His speech was coherent and his ideas well-connected. I saw no evidence of clinical depression. His mannerisms were appropriate. His thought processes were sharp and well-formulated. No indication of delusionary thought or impaired judgment. His memory was surprisingly good for a man his age . . .

STACIE: The only word *I* could remember was *hippopotamus.*

KIM: Yeah. He was alert, oriented, articulate. And to be honest, he was right about how the only reason his decision was being questioned is because we have the power to override it . . . well, that and the fact that we think it's a bad decision.

STACIE: Actually, I'm not so sure I do. If I were in his position, I don't know that *I'd* want to risk winding up with the interventions he's liable to need and not being in control. He's certainly got a point about letting nature take its course and all. I've already seen enough patients to last me who kept getting pulled back every time they were ready to go. And for what? Still, I don't feel very comfortable about putting a DNR order on his chart on a Friday night just before Christmas without being able to talk with any of his family or even Dr. Raphael. But it's what Mr. Bitone wants. So unless you think there's some reason to doubt his mental status, I guess that's what I'll do.

KIM: Nope. I think you're right. It's *his* decision. I just hope nothin' happens. Anyway, I gotta go. I'll dictate my consult note later tonight. Good luck.

STACIE: Thanks a lot for coming over. I know you didn't need this.

KIM: Actually, it was pretty interesting. It'll give me something to think about tonight. And he is a sweet old guy. I'll see you later.

STACIE: Bye.

(As Kim walks away, Stacie turns back and heads toward the ICU.)

RICHARD: So, what's the verdict?

STACIE: It's not like that at all. I just needed to get a second opinion. I'm still in training, you know . . . and I just don't want to do anything that might hurt you. (*Moving the pages around on her clipboard, Stacie stands, leaning a little against the foot of Richard's bed.*) Well, I've got a DNR form here. You do understand that if you sign this it means that if your heart should stop, for any reason at all, we wouldn't try to resuscitate you?

(*Richard nods as Stacie looks at him inquiringly.*) Because of your condition we're going to have to notify your next of kin that you've been made DNR. But unless you went into arrest when your wife was actually here, we wouldn't have time to call anyone, and legally we wouldn't be allowed to intervene to resuscitate you. (*Stacie waits, but Richard doesn't say anything.*) It means that if your heart stops you'd die.

(*There is silence for a few moments, then Richard speaks quietly.*)

RICHARD: I know.

STACIE: (*concerned and rather uncomfortable*) OK. Just so long as you understand what this means. And you're sure you want this done tonight?

RICHARD: Uh-huh.

STACIE: OK. Read this over, and if you have any questions be *sure* to ask. I'll wait until you're done. (*Stacie stands at Richard's bed as patiently as she can. She watches him reading, then looks up at his heart monitor. His heartbeat is 82 and steady. After a few minutes Richard looks up as he lays the DNR form on his lap. Stacie waits and then somewhat apprehensively asks*) No questions?

RICHARD: Nope.

STACIE: OK, then, just sign there at the bottom and I'll make sure everything gets taken care of in terms of your chart. If you change your mind, be sure to tell one of the nurses and they'll let me know so I can change the orders.

RICHARD: I'll let you know.

STACIE: Alright. Well . . . good night.

RICHARD: Good night. See you in the morning.

STACIE: (*walking away, she says quietly to herself*) I certainly hope so.

(*Stacie goes to the nurses' station and makes a copy of the DNR form that Richard has signed. She then attaches the copy to Richard's chart and places the original in the designated file drawer. It's about 10:45 and so rather than have to explain the situation twice, Stacie waits until the night shift of nurses comes on duty at 11:00 before communicating Richard's DNR order to the staff who will oversee his care until 7:00 the next morning. As the nurses are busy, no one questions Stacie to any great extent about the timing or nature of the DNR order. Stacie then goes back to the doctors' lounge and, after trying unsuccessfully to read for a while, goes to bed around midnight. At about 7:15 Stacie, who has already begun her ward rounds, is paged by the ICU. Stacie returns the call immediately. She is then told that Richard Bitone is having a major MI and is asked by one of the nurses to authorize life-saving intervention, effectively overriding the DNR order.*)

STACIE: Don't do anything! I'll be there in less than a minute.

(*Stacie runs full sprint to the ICU and finds three nurses around Richard's bed. Sara is starting a second IV, two other nurses have the crash cart unpacked. Ready and waiting are syringes filled with epinephrine and lidocaine, a ventilation bag, an intubation kit, and a defibrillator. Stacie pulls up, breathless, and surveys the situation. The heart monitor shows a flat line with a heart rate of 0.*)

SARA: (*hurriedly*) It just stopped about ten seconds ago!

STACIE: (*panting*) He has a DNR order. We can't do anything.

SARA: But he'll die!

STACIE: (*still surveying the situation*) I know. But that's what he wanted.

SARA: Who authorized the DNR order?!

STACIE: (*now a little more collected and resolved to see the situation through*) I did—last night. I also spoke with Dr. Pearlman, and he understood the situation.

SARA: Does Betty know?

STACIE: No.

SARA: Don't you think she ought to know about this?!

STACIE: Ideally, yes. But this isn't the time for that. And anyhow, I don't know how to get in touch with her. She's off visiting some relatives for the weekend.

SARA: (*not able to believe what she's hearing*) So you're just going to let him die?!!

STACIE: (*sadly*) I don't have any choice. That's what he wanted.

SARA: And what are you gonna tell his wife?

STACIE: The truth. What else?

SARA: (*very angrily*) I am *not* responsible for this!! And I'm going to register my objection and file a complaint with our supervisor! This isn't right. You don't just let people die because sometime late at night when they were tired they told you not to save them! I'm tellin' you right now, this isn't right!! (*Sara stares hard at Stacie. Seeing that Stacie is not going to change her decision to let Richard die, Sara looks at Richard and then glares at Stacie.*) You're the doctor!

(*Stacie stands at the foot of the bed as Sara and the two nurses clean up the crash cart. The two other nurses are quiet and almost demure. After they leave, Stacie remains. She stares at the flat EKG, waits for a few minutes, and then checks Richard's pulse and respiration to certify that he is dead. Stacie then informs the nurses that Richard has died and will need to be taken care of. Stacie continues her morning rounds on her remaining patients. At 9:00 Sta-*

cie learns that Betty has called and been told of her husband's death. Stacie is told that Betty will be arriving sometime midafternoon. Stacie then calls Dr. Mark Pearlman at home, explains what has happened, and asks if he'd be willing to stay on after his rounds so that Stacie doesn't have to deal with Betty all by herself. Mark says he would and that he'll be in around 10:00. Stacie is waiting when Mark arrives.)

MARK: Tough morning, huh?

STACIE: Toughest one I've had in a while, Dr. Pearlman. And I don't think the afternoon is going to be any better. Why does this kind of thing always happen just when you're almost done? Another two days and I'd've been outta here.

MARK: Well . . . as Charlton Heston said, what's done is done and can't be undone.

STACIE: I guess so. I just don't know what I'm going to tell his wife. I feel like I had to let him die . . . at least if I was going to respect his autonomy. He knew what to expect, there was no reason to think that his mental status was impaired in any way, this is what he wanted. *(shaking her head slowly)* I just wish he had talked to his wife about it first. She's gonna think I killed him. That's what Sara down in ICU thinks. She said she's going to file a complaint. *(Stacie sighs and swallows hard.)*

MARK: Well, from what you told me, you did everything right. No one ever said that the right thing couldn't also be tragic. Let's start rounds, and then later when Mrs. Bitone comes in I'll give you a call. Just make sure you have all the paperwork . . . and if you can, have Kim Bodle write up a report of her assessment of Mr. Bitone. That'll help . . . cheer up, this is what medicine's about—doing the right thing even when it hurts.

⑤ The Future of Autonomy

To establish, as I hope to, that autonomous patients' PSR decisions should be respected by HCPs, three issues still need to be addressed. The first is whether concern for a patient's future autonomy or future selves can override the importance of respecting her present autonomous decisions. Second, we must somehow reconcile how a patient's greatly imprudent decisions can yet be seen as autonomous. Third, and perhaps most importantly, we must discuss whether respecting autonomous PSR decisions has sufficient value to override competing concerns. I will turn now to the first of these projects.

For any given patient, future autonomy refers to a future state of being, which, should it come about, may describe a single point in time, periods of time, or even the whole of that patient's future autonomous existence. Clearly, there is no necessary opposition between future autonomy and the present exercise of autonomy, and in fact many (present) autonomous decisions take the preservation and furtherance of an autonomous existence to be a fundamental interest that ought to be promoted. Nonetheless, in many cases present autonomous decisions conflict with the interests of preserving or promoting future autonomy, and one must choose between the two. This situation is perhaps most pressing when autonomous actions are greatly imprudent and likely to compromise future well-being in addition to autonomy. Of course, it is a real and important question whether greatly imprudent actions *can* be autonomous.[1] But for the time being, I will assume that an action *can* be both autonomous and imprudent and that it does make sense to speak of Alan's refusal of a lumbar puncture as a present autonomous imprudent decision, in direct conflict with both future well-being and the prospect of future autonomy. What, then, are the arguments for opposing such actions, for promoting future autonomy over and against the present exercise of autonomy?

The most frequently advanced arguments are utilitarian and are generally based on well-being. They argue that it is legitimate and justifiable to override Sally's present autonomous decisions to promote her future autonomy *if* doing so would maximize Sally's well-being. Though less com-

mon, some consequentialist arguments alternatively propose that autonomy, as a commodity, should be maximized. A second genre of argument
supposes that we have a responsibility not to wrong our "future selves." Of
the various ways to ground such a claim,[2] arguably the most plausible is advanced by Derek Parfit, who relies on the larger claim that what matters is
not personal identity, but psychological connectedness.[3]

The utilitarian argument based on well-being is not really an argument
about future autonomy at all. Rather, it is simply the traditional utilitarian
argument that the right course of action is that which maximizes happiness or well-being. As such, it is open to a number of standard responses,
two of which are particularly persuasive here. First, this utilitarian thesis
cannot acknowledge that exercising autonomy has any value beyond its
contribution to well-being. But because many of us believe that autonomous action can be and often is important and meaningful *irrespective* of
its contribution to well-being, such a narrow gauge of value is alone
sufficient to defeat the utilitarian argument.[4] Second, the very presumption
that well-being can be maximized begs the question, Who will carry out the
calculation, and according to whose standards for well-being? Moreover, by
what process will these standards be formed? Arguably, no universally accepted criteria for settling these questions exist. But if utilitarianism cannot avoid significant reference to self-governance at some level, then it is
not at all clear how autonomy is being superseded by well-being. A third
and fairly powerful response is that well-being probably could not be maximized if autonomous PSR decisions were continually subject to being
trumped. Hence even utilitarians should adopt the rule that autonomous
PSR decisions should be respected.

In contrast with the utilitarian argument for well-being, the consequentialist argument for maximizing autonomy and the future selves argument
each present a more genuine conflict between present and future autonomy. In both instances at issue is the relative importance of, on the one hand,
Sally's exercising present autonomy and, on the other hand, preserving Sally's future capacity for autonomy. Since the degree of risk as well as the actual amount of future autonomy at stake will vary from case to case, it is
unlikely that either argument will prefer future autonomy unconditionally.
Nonetheless, I want to resist the conclusion that it is *ever* right to override
Sally's present autonomous decisions to promote her future autonomy.

One response to the consequentialist position that one's future capacity
for autonomy should be maximized at the expense of one's present exercise of autonomy is John Dewey's claim that to sacrifice the present for the
future is to empty the present of all meaning.[5] Clearly, we must understand

"sacrificing the present for the future" as something more than merely making a sacrifice now to secure some future gain, for we all do that. Sacrificing the present for the future involves uncoupling ends and means in such a way that one's present activities no longer reflect the principles that ground one's values, upon which one's priorities, and in that sense "meaning," are based. Thus, one "sacrifices the present" when one renders present activity a mere instrumentality by abandoning ultimate principles, albeit for the sake of some future state. This first response, then, is that by failing to respect Sally's autonomous PSR decisions we sacrifice the value that being autonomous brings to Sally. This forfeiture involves not only the value we ascribe to her as an autonomous being but also the value Sally ascribes to herself. The strength of this response depends greatly on how convincing are the arguments for the importance of being autonomous. But to the extent that one is convinced that being autonomous is fundamental for ascribing value and meaning to individuals, this Deweyan response is quite telling.

Still, one might argue that this response is mistaken in that it conflates two distinct senses of autonomy. For while her *capacity* for autonomy allows us to ascribe certain fundamental values to Sally, one may yet deny that this is in any way compromised when we fail to respect the *exercise* of autonomous preferences. Thus, for the Deweyan response to succeed, it must be shown that it is problematic to value autonomy as a capacity and yet fail to respect the exercise of that capacity.

This challenge can be taken in either of two ways, depending on whether the present capacity or the future capacity for autonomy is being juxtaposed with the present exercise of autonomy. If it is present capacity, I respond that it is hard to understand how one's actions can be based on the value of Sally's present capacity to be autonomous and yet fail to respect the exercise of that capacity in PSR matters. For what could it mean to value the present capacity without also valuing its present exercise? One would need somehow to establish that the concept of being self-governing has value apart from its instantiation, that is, the act of being self-governing. But beyond perhaps some aesthetic appreciation, what is left? Apart from its exercise, what can ground the value we place in the present capacity for autonomy? If not its exercise, what can explain the importance we attribute to being autonomous, its foundational role in creating value and meaning?[6] There may be many good reasons not to respect Sally's present autonomous decisions—harm to others, violation of contracts, and so forth. But if we are acting *out of respect for* Sally's present capacity for autonomy, it seems disingenuous to believe that her present autonomous decisions (which exercise involves her deciding the meaning and importance of her own interconnections with the world) do not also warrant respect.[7]

But does the same relation exist between acting out of respect for Sally's future capacity for autonomy and respecting the present exercise of autonomy? Presumably, one can value a future state as distinct from its realization, as one may value the capacity for motherhood apart from any particular instantiation of being a mother. But with regard to autonomy the question is whether the value attributed to autonomy can be located in the future capacity as distinct from its present exercise. To begin, there is no reason to think that being autonomous at some future point is more valuable than being autonomous now, just as there is no reason to think that exercising autonomy at some future time is more valuable than exercising it now. But, moreover, there is reason to think that what makes autonomy meaningful and of central importance is its instantiation in the present. For without some realization of autonomy there would be nothing but "the idea" of self-governance, nothing but a future state without grounding, without substance, without consequences. Without some actual instantiation of autonomy it is hard to know what it could mean to genuinely value autonomy. For being autonomous, that is, living an autonomous existence, could no longer be held up as central to the value ascribed to autonomy. But if this is so, then it seems to defeat the claim that we can locate autonomy's meaning and central importance in the future capacity for autonomy, in which case it is problematic to use "regard for future autonomy" to trump the present exercise of autonomy. As Dewey understood, in a sense the present is all we have, and as such it must be the locus of meaning and value and the focus of our attention.

Of course, one might accept the above arguments and yet claim they neither reflect nor address the central conflict between the exercise of present autonomy and maximizing patients' future capacity for autonomy. That is, one might claim that the consequentialist position is not that the meaning and importance of autonomy reside somewhere other than in its present exercise, but rather that given the importance of exercising autonomy we ought to maximize such "present exercises," or at least the number of opportunities for such exercise. There are two responses to this charge, one direct, the other indirect.

The indirect response is that while larger amounts of, or opportunities for, autonomous decisions often may be a good thing, it is not the quantity of autonomous decisions (even over a lifetime) that secures autonomy its place within our value scheme, but the *nature* of autonomous behavior and of living an autonomous existence. The autonomous wish of a dying man is no less valuable for his having a short time to live. Nor is there a direct relationship between the value of our autonomous decisions and the extent to which they (subsequently) affect the autonomous nature of our lives—many acclaimed autonomous decisions happen to involve significant sacrifice of subsequent opportunities to exercise autonomy, if not sacrifice of the capacity for autonomy itself. Moreover, it is at the very least arguable whether increasing the amount that Sally exercises her autonomy contributes to the value of her life. Just as a story may be better constructed and more meaningful for having less words, one's life may be better or even more valuable for having a smaller number of autonomous decisions. While this reasoning does not establish that we should never maximize opportunities for exercising autonomy, it ought to be clear that the consequentialist maxim is inadequate to serve as either a general criterion for guiding action or as a means for differentiating appropriate from inappropriate actions.

A more direct response speaks to the consequentialist's claim that the exercise of autonomy is being promoted and that at stake in overriding the present exercise of autonomy is simply a small segment of a much larger picture. Clearly such a scenario is consistent with promoting other sorts of goods. For example, one can promote well-being by administering a drug that makes a patient worse off, but in the interest of making her better. In so acting one promotes well-being, acts from the motive of promoting well-being, and yet intentionally undermines well-being in the process. The question is whether it is possible to override the exercise of autonomy *while acting out of respect for* the exercise of autonomy. I contend that it is not possible, and that the difference is rooted in the fact that, unlike respect for autonomy, there are different senses in which one can understand well-being. It is not incompatible with respecting well-being to believe that overall well-being can involve discomfort, pain, anxiety, or even minor physiologic demise. If Sally has an emotionally painful experience, we say that she deals with it in a healthy way when she confronts it, even when confronting it is difficult and involves pain. Because our notion of well-being shifts in terms of its frame of reference, sometimes being larger, sometimes narrower, there is (only) apparent contradiction when two frames of reference are included in one instance. The apparent contradiction is really just a difference in perspective.[8]

The same cannot be said regarding respect for autonomy. There is no sense in which I can be *acting out of respect for* your exercise of autonomy and at the same time undermining your present exercise of autonomy. For at that moment I cannot say there is some larger sense of *your exercise* of autonomy that I am respecting. There is no larger frame of reference for my respect beyond your exercise of autonomy right there and then. Now, this is not to say that I am not acting so as to maximize the number of opportunities for exercising autonomy, for indeed that is my intention. Nor does it deny that maximizing the number of opportunities for exercising autonomy is, in and of itself, a laudable goal. But many actions are inappropriate despite their laudable goals. It is in fact a general problem that consequentialist analyses cannot distinguish between legitimate and illegitimate means for maximizing desired ends.

I have argued that there is something fundamental about regarding individuals as autonomous and that one cannot act out of respect for their autonomy without respecting their present exercise of autonomy. Additionally, I have argued that the value of an autonomous existence is not determined by the number of opportunities one has for exercising autonomy. One might seek to maximize Sally's opportunities for exercising autonomy without regard for its effect on her present exercise of autonomy.[9] But this would not be consistent with *acting out of respect for* autonomy. Put simply, "respect for autonomy" cannot be used to justify overriding the present exercise of autonomy.[10]

Future Selves

Another attempted justification for subjugating the exercise of present autonomy to future interests involves "concern for future selves." One version of this rather perplexing view is advanced by Parfit, who argues that because it is psychological connectedness and not physical identity that matters, future selves may stand apart from prior selves to the extent that they are less psychologically connected. In Parfit's view one has a responsibility not to commit one's future selves to that which it is wrong to commit others. And he goes on to argue that one stands to future selves in a special relation that entails special obligations—such as one has to one's parents, children, pupils, patients, clients, or constituents.[11] Thus, when Sally acts in greatly imprudent ways the wrongness of her imprudence is not excused by the fact that the outcome will be worse only for her. The notion is that Sally's future self would be irrevocably committed to things that would be to her detriment, and while Sally could do this to *herself,* she could not do it to others, and Sally's future self stands as an "other" to her present self.

Clearly Parfit's position challenges individual sovereignty over PSR matters. For to the extent that future selves do stand apart from prior selves, there is less of a qualitative distinction differentiating Sally from other concerned parties with regard to decisions that affect Sally's future selves. In other words, because not just Sally but others can be competent guardians for (and have an interest in) Sally's future selves, decision-making is no longer the sole prerogative of Sally's prior self, that is, no longer the sole prerogative of Sally. In fact, Parfit writes that because future selves have no vote their interests need to be protected. In this way others' paternalistic interests regarding Sally's future selves come to be seen as a form of public interest similar to the interest society exercises for children over and against less than diligent parents.

Both practical and theoretical responses to this kind of challenge rebut the claim that concern for future selves will or should override an autonomous individual's prerogative to have final say over PSR decisions. First, because compared to other potential decision-makers Sally generally will have more extensive knowledge of what is in the best interests of her future selves, those interests will be best protected and respected by deferring to Sally's own decisions. Second, seldom will psychological connectedness be so dissociated that it will make sense to promote Sally's future autonomy over her present exercise of autonomy. That is, in the vast majority of cases Sally's future self will be sufficiently connected to her present self that it will not be appropriate to regard that future self as an "other." Sally's present self seldom will stand as just another helpful bystander with the responsibility to protect the interests of her future selves. Third, if Parfit is right that Sally is barred from committing (sufficiently disconnected) future selves to irrevocable conditions, especially commitments that are likely to be detrimental,[12] the same argument should apply to other major life decisions, such as having children, going into massive debt for a purchase, undergoing plastic surgery, or becoming a professional boxer. Presumably, much turns upon how "greatly imprudent" is defined, for certainly imprudent actions vary in degree. Additionally, Parfit refers to the steepness of the discount rate, that is, the degree to which future suffering can be offset by present pleasures. Nevertheless, even conservative cost-benefit analyses would likely judge all sorts of everyday activities "morally wrong," from smoking cigarettes to having "unsafe sex" to heroic acts that place one in great danger. Parfit writes that the truth may be disturbing. But the ramifications of his claim that greatly imprudent actions are morally wrong would be more than disturbing. Who could legitimately make these major, risky life decisions? Could we make them at all?

Fourth, even when Sally's future selves *do* stand apart, it is odd to regard these future selves as needing protection from Sally. For we know that any future self must evolve from Sally and so will seldom possess its own distinct values and interests. If one is looking to "build in" to a future self some "objective" set of standards to gauge the reasonability of Sally's decisions, such standards already can be found in the normative qualifications necessary for having the capacity for autonomy. Of course, one might counter this by claiming that "autonomy does not include the right to impose upon oneself, *for no good reason,* great harm."[13] But, as even Parfit admits, it is problematic who should determine what counts as "for no good reason." If a man with early stage testicular cancer refuses hormonal or surgical therapy because of their "emasculating" effects, was there good enough reason? If a woman chooses to have silicone breast implants to please her boyfriend, was there good enough reason? So long as a person satisfies the normative qualifications necessary to qualify as autonomous, who is to judge for that person what counts as a reasonable trade-off? To justify overriding Sally's PSR decisions out of concern for her future selves, there must be some nonarbitrary rationale for making such judgments, but at present such a rationale seems rather elusive.

Finally, suppose we did come to regard future selves as the children of present selves, children whose interests stood apart and required safeguarding.[14] Presumably, PSR decisions that "unreasonably" compromised the "objective" interests and opportunities of future selves, placing future selves at great risk, could be overridden. But this would include decisions whose "unreasonableness" was rooted in the very individuality of a prior self's (idiosyncratic) interests. And surely this is too extreme; it would place greater restrictions on prior selves than we place on the parents of real children. Although society acknowledges a general set of interests and opportunities that ought to "belong" to children and be protected, we do not thereby restrict parents' PSR decisions on that basis alone. Imagine a Jewish couple, the De la Steinbergs, in fifteenth-century Spain who refuses to convert to Christianity and thereby commits their three-month-old child to innumerable disadvantages and misfortunes. I doubt the general set of interests and opportunities society might wish to protect for that child includes any commitment to Judaism. But in the absence of such specific commitments and interests (which seems a reasonable assumption), if we applied the same criteria proposed for future selves we would have to conclude that the need to protect the interests of their child would justify overriding the De la Steinbergs' decision not to convert. No doubt many cases are more problematic—for example, pregnant women who injure their fetuses by choosing to abuse drugs. But in plenty of cases we do not regard injury to a child's interests and reduction of her opportunities as sufficient grounds for restricting parents' PSR decisions. I would argue that it is at the very least counterintuitive to think that we should place restrictions on actions out of concern for future selves that we would not place on parents out of concern for wholly distinct human beings. We avoid such a conclusion if we reject the notion that future selves have a disconnected, "objective" set of values that must be protected. But if we do reject this tenet and recognize that the interests of future selves are intimately linked with the prior autonomous self, any basis for protecting future selves from the interests of the prior self vanishes. And thus there is no future-regarding basis for overriding an individual's prerogative to have final say over autonomous PSR decisions.

This is not say, however, that future selves deserve no consideration. Surely, there is no disrespect in having concern for how an individual's future life will go, as well as the sort of person she will develop into. That is only natural. How strange it would seem to profess genuine regard for another but to have no concern whatsoever beyond her most immediate, present existence. And yet it can be quite difficult to manifest concern for future selves while also respecting the sovereignty of the present autonomous self (in PSR matters)—not only because it requires great sensitivity but also because respecting autonomous choices may involve tragic consequences. The following case illustrates that to effect these dual goals of concern and respect one must be prepared both to work very hard—at understanding and practical reasoning—and to take risks whose consequences can be far reaching and tragic.

Dialogue 4: Protecting Respect

Herman Lawrence grew up in Pittsburgh but moved away during the Great Depression to find work. He lied about his age and experience and in 1935 was able to get a job as a steelworker in San Francisco. Herman spent the war repairing ships and by the end of World War II had married and bought a house just west of Golden Gate Park, "out in the avenues" as the locals would say. It was there that he helped raise his family and continues now to live a quiet existence. Though himself the second oldest of six children, at seventy-three years of age Herman is the only member of his immediate family still alive. Two brothers died of heart attacks, one at forty-eight, the other at forty-nine. One sister was killed in an auto accident, another sister died of colon cancer at age fifty-one, and Herman's youngest brother died just last year of lung cancer at age fifty-eight. Cancer also killed both of Herman's parents some thirty years ago. Herman's own health has been relatively good despite various minor work-related accidents and some arthritis from his years of physical labor. Herman is about twenty-five pounds overweight, thanks in part to his love for his wife's Italian cooking, but otherwise has remained free of any major injury or disease. Yet the succession of deaths in his family along with the natural aging process have progressively chipped away at Herman's sense of well-being, and over the last twenty years Herman has become increasingly worried about his health. Herman has dealt with these worries by attempting to avoid confronting anything that might be considered a threat to his health. The primary form this has taken is denial.

For the past twenty years Herman as well as his wife and children have had Dr. Albert Bang as their physician. A second-generation Chinese American, Albert was born and raised in San Francisco and received all his medical training in the Bay Area. Albert, who is sixty-three, has come to know Herman and his family rather well over the years, and likes them a great deal. Albert has recently been joined in his practice by his son, Dr. Robert Bang, who just finished his residency in family practice. Robert, who is thirty-one, has joined his father with the understanding that over the next few years he will gradually take over the care of his father's patients. Albert and Robert have a very good working and personal relationship. It is easy to see that they enjoy each other's company and have a great deal of respect for one another. Over the past twelve months Robert has been introduced to virtually all his father's patients, and most of them are now comfortable being treated by either Dr. Bang.

It is now early July and the two Drs. Bang are discussing what to do with Herman Lawrence. Herman has been troubled by what he describes as mild abdominal pain. Though this pain began in mid-April, it was not until more than a month later that Herman was finally coaxed by his wife, Linda, to have it checked out. Herman was seen at that time by the younger Dr. Bang, to whom he explained that the pain "wasn't any big deal." Robert did an initial workup and found nothing conclusive. After consulting with his father, Robert decided that Herman's discomfort was likely due to increased stomach acid and that a few weeks of H2–blockers would probably do the trick. By mid-June, however, Herman still was not feeling any better, and so it was decided that, given the strong family history for cancer, a more extensive workup should be done. The results of this workup have just come in. According to the pathology report and the radionuclide scans, Herman Lawrence has a grade B1 cancer of the descending colon.

ROBERT: Well, it could've been worse. Since it's grade B1, the cancer hasn't gotten out of the muscularis yet. They'll have to resect part of the bowel along with some para- and epicolic nodes, but he's really lucky; it's unlikely there's any involvement of the primary lymph nodes, much less any metastases to the liver. It's a good thing we caught it this early; there's a lot that still can be done at this stage in the game.

ALBERT: True enough. But it's going to be tough going getting him into treatment.

ROBERT: What do you mean?

ALBERT: I mean that Herman Lawrence may look like your average patient. But he has a depressive streak that runs the length of his medical chart.

ROBERT: I'm sorry, Dad, I still don't follow you.

ALBERT: Remember during your second year in medical school I told you about this patient who I had to send for counseling before I could remove what turned out to be a benign dermatofibroma? Well, this is the guy.

ROBERT: What's the story? Why's he so . . . ?

ALBERT: You knew that he's got a strong family history for cancer?

ROBERT: Uh-huh.

ALBERT: Well, he's the only one left. Both his parents, a sister, and his youngest brother all died of cancer. Different kinds, but cancer just the same. And it doesn't help anything that his two other brothers had fatal heart attacks before the age of fifty and that his other sister died on the operating table after a head-on car crash. Just the *idea* of being sick makes him ill. (*Robert groans, though he's actually come to enjoy his father's bad puns.*) It's like death is something he simply can't deal with.

ROBERT: But I thought you said he was a steelworker or something?

ALBERT: He was! Used to hang off girders hundreds of feet in the air. He was one of those guys that helped build the Golden Gate Bridge back in the thirties. He says heights don't bother him . . . ugh! . . . makes the soles of my feet tingle just thinking about it. I guess it's just something about being sick, just scares him practically to death.

ROBERT: Hmph. How odd. Is his wife like that, too?

ALBERT: Not at all. She's the paradigm of a rational thinker. They really make quite a pair.

ROBERT: How do you tell him bad news? Especially something like this. If a dermatofibroma requires counseling, what is this going to do to him?

ALBERT: Well, I don't expect it'll be easy. But my guess is that if we go through Linda, his wife, she'll figure out something to tell him so that we don't wind up beating him over the head with it. Yup, I'd say discussing this with him was medically contraindicated.

ROBERT: Do you mean to say that you don't want me to tell him his own test results?

ALBERT: Not unless you feel like adding a psychiatric consult to all this.

ROBERT: I find it hard to believe that he'd really get as bad as all that. He doesn't look that fragile.

ALBERT: Well, looks can be deceiving.

ROBERT: I don't know, Dad . . . it doesn't seem right. How's he supposed to make an informed decision if he doesn't know what he's got?

ALBERT: Well, hopefully Linda will be able to do something. I suggest we give her a call and meet with her first. Then, maybe you and the two of them can get together later in the week to sort out his treatment.

ROBERT: This doesn't seem right to me. In the first place, we don't have a right to divulge information about *his* health without *his* permission. And in the second place, it seems pretty paternalistic to think that he won't be able to handle the information. It's not like he's a little kid or anything. You've known him and his wife a lot longer than I have. But I don't think we'd be justified in withholding relevant medical information from him unless he's given us unambiguous directives *not* to tell him. Do you see what I mean?

ALBERT: Robert, you need to understand that this isn't some abstract ethics discussion here. We're talking about Herman Lawrence, someone I've known for twenty years. We're talking about a particular individual and what's best for him.

ROBERT: Dad, it's not our decision to make. I'm not saying we should call him in and say, "Hey, by the way, you've got cancer like the rest of your family. What do you want to do about it?" But I think we're on really shaky ground, ethically that is, if we start making decisions about what he should and shouldn't know about his own health. And I don't think it's much better to let his wife decide, either. We have a responsibility to respect his autonomy. And that means giving him the information, albeit sensitively.

ALBERT: But if he doesn't want it?

ROBERT: Well, we don't know that.

ALBERT: What I'm trying to say is that I *know* Herman Lawrence. Herman is not the kind of man who wants to know he's got cancer. If he's got to go into the hospital for an operation, which he does, then he's not going to want to know that the reason he's going in is because he has cancer. It wouldn't make any difference that it's an early stage cancer or that he's got an 85 percent five-year survival rate with an operation and an 80 percent chance of complete cure. *Cancer* is simply not a word he wants to hear.

ROBERT: What would you tell him?

ALBERT: We could tell him he's got a colonic neoplasia or something. We could refer him to my old friend, Dr. Lo—he does great work on these things. He trained at the U of C under what's-his-name. Anyway, if we talked to Linda about it first, I really don't think there'd be any problem. We could explain to Herman all the risks of surgery and use medical terminology so that Herman wouldn't know it was cancer. And then just have him sign the consent form. Herman's an extreme case. But you'd be surprised how often you have to coddle patients. A lot of 'em just don't want to know.

ROBERT: I don't mean to be insulting, Dad, but things have changed since you trained in medicine. You can't just disregard patients' autonomy like that.

ALBERT: I'm not as out of touch as you think. I get the *Hastings Center Report* and *JAMA* and the *New England Journal.* I've read about autonomy. But if what you really value is Herman Lawrence's autonomy, then you have to realize that by telling him that he's got cancer you're gonna literally destroy his autonomy. He'll go into a tailspin, and you'll never see his autonomy again. Certainly he'll never be the same. If you don't believe me, then you can talk to his wife. But she won't tell you anything different than I did.

ROBERT: Look, let's assume just for the sake of argument that you're right, that if we tell Herman that he's got cancer he'll go into a true clinical depression. I still say that we need to find out from him whether he *wants* to know about his condition. It may well be that he tells us "no," that we should just do what we think is right, and he'll ask us when he wants to know about something. I don't have any problem with that. But if he wants to know, that's *his* decision. And it's not our business, it's not even his wife's business, to keep that from him. People make bad decisions all the time. We'd just be using the power we have to keep him from making a bad decision. But it's his decision and he has the right to make it. I mean, if he's as bad as you say, then surely he'd know enough not to want to know whether or not he had cancer, right?

ALBERT: I think you're oversimplifying this. People don't fit that neatly into the kinds of ethical arguments you're making. You can't just ask someone whether they want to know whether or not they have cancer. It doesn't work that way. You go by a person's habits, by what you know about them. There's a lot more to people than what they *say.* That's one thing you'll learn as you get more experience with patients. You really have to learn to read between the lines.

ROBERT: Dad, you talk like you're some kind of soothsayer. You can't ever know what's going on in someone else's head. For all you know, Herman Lawrence may well overcome his fear if he's forced to confront it head-on. By making this decision for him you're denying him that chance, the chance to develop.

ALBERT: That may be. But that's a different argument. Let's assume, like you said before, that I am right. Let's assume that if Herman Lawrence finds out that he has cancer he'll enter a dark cloud and possibly never come out. Part of the reason he and his wife have come to me for twenty years is that they know that I'll do what's in their best interest. They trust me. That's why I'm still their doctor.

ROBERT: I'm not saying they don't trust you *or* that they shouldn't. All I'm saying is that I don't think that you, or his wife, have a right to decide what he should and shouldn't be able to deal with. Doesn't *he* have the right to decide what he's capable of? It's one thing to say that we should talk with his wife about the best way to talk with Herman regarding his health. That has to do with strategy. But it's quite another thing to say that we, or his wife, should be deciding for him what he should know or what he should do. He must know that he doesn't deal well with health problems. Are you telling me he doesn't even have the capacity to decide how he *wants* to handle stuff like this?

ALBERT: You lost me.

ROBERT: What I mean is that Herman isn't oblivious to his inability to deal with health-related problems. So in that sense he understands that when he's up against some problem that threatens his sense of well-being he needs to find some way of dealing with it.

ALBERT: And what I'm telling you is that the way he deals with it is by shutting off.

ROBERT: I understand that. But surely we can approach the issue in a way that allows him to stay in the conversation, if only to delegate decision-making to his wife, or even us. What I'm saying is that to assume that Herman should have no role in deciding how some aspect of his life as serious as what we're dealing with here will be managed is to treat him like a, like a little kid who isn't capable of running his own life—and that isn't right. If you want me to call his wife and speak with her about how best to deal with Herman, I'm willing to do that. But I don't think we can make a decision without input from Herman. And to tell you the truth, I don't think I'm comfortable telling his wife that he has cancer before he has the opportunity to know and understand his situation. I mean,

Herman may not even want his wife to know about this. I'm willing to talk with her, but at some level it's Herman that needs to decide.

ALBERT: I don't think that's a good idea.

ROBERT: (*uncomfortable, but resolute*) I sense that we've reached an impasse here. (*Robert waits for his father to say something, but Albert just stands quietly, his hands clasped in front of him, pensively biting at his lower lip.*) Well . . . (*Robert smiles and gives his father a questioning look*) unless you're planning on pulling rank, I'm going to do this in the way that I think is right. I'll give his wife a call, ask her to come in, tell her about our concerns— without telling her that it's cancer or that he needs an operation—and then work out with her a way of dealing with him. Can you live with that?

ALBERT: This is *your* patient, at least for this go-round. So I won't tell you what to do. But I would like to be there when you meet with Linda. I think she's going to have a hard time with the way you want to handle this. If you want my advice, I think it's important that you *really listen* to Linda. She's the one who's going to have to deal with Herman for the rest of his life, not you. I won't intervene. But if she asks, I'll say what I think. OK?

(*Robert calls Linda Lawrence at home and they arrange for her to come in at 5:30 that afternoon while her husband goes over to the park to sit and talk with his buddies. Linda explains that this is not a problem since they weren't planning to eat until 8:00 anyway. When Linda arrives she is seated in Robert's office. After a few minutes the two Drs. Bang enter the room and as Linda watches them come in together she is struck by how similar their mannerisms are. As Robert sits at his desk across from Linda, Albert takes a seat next to her and moves it so that he can view both Linda and his son.*)

ROBERT: Sorry to keep you waiting. I was in with someone and . . . well, sometimes patients really like to know what's going on with them . . .

LINDA: That's alright. I wasn't waiting long. You know, the two of you really look remarkably alike . . .

ALBERT: (*joking*) Well, I should hope so! (*Robert shakes his head, wondering where his father gets it.*) But thanks just the same. It's always a pleasure to see you.

LINDA: Thank you, Dr. Bang. It's always good to see you, too. (*Linda pauses, then says a little nervously*) So . . . was there something you wanted to talk with me about?

ROBERT: Yes there was.

(*As Robert speaks Linda turns to him. She is a little surprised, having expected that she would be dealing with the elder Dr. Bang.*)

ROBERT: Um, you know that your husband has been having some abdominal pain. At first we thought it might just be too much acid, but the medicine we gave him didn't seem to help. That's why a week or so ago we arranged for a more extensive work-up. The reason I wanted to speak with you is that we received the results from those tests today . . . annnnnd, w-we think that your husband is going to need some . . . well, some follow-up treatment. (*Linda begins to look very worried and looks to Albert for some sort of relief or reassurance. Albert doesn't say anything or make any gestures, and Robert continues.*) In speaking with my father, he explained to me that Herman doesn't do very well when he's confronted with . . . certain health problems. And so what I'd like to talk with you about is how best to go about discussing this issue with your husband.

LINDA: What does he have? What's the matter with him?

ROBERT: Because I haven't yet discussed the results with your husband, I don't feel I can divulge that information. I . . .

LINDA: (*turning to Albert, confused*) What does he mean?

ROBERT: (*Robert gently continues, causing Linda to turn back to him*) I mean that patient confidentiality requires that I not discuss a patient's medical condition until the patient has been consulted.

LINDA: (*confused, and not used to this at all when having dealt with Albert*) But I'm his *wife*. Why shouldn't I know? We've been married for over forty years. (*Again, Linda looks to Albert for relief.*)

ALBERT: (*to Robert*) May I?

ROBERT: (*a little relieved by his father's intervention*) Please.

ALBERT: What Robert means, Linda, is that he thinks that Herman is going to have to deal with this situation. And what Robert wants is for you to help us figure out how best to discuss Herman's situation and options *with* Herman.

LINDA: But how can I do that unless I know what's the matter with him? You know how Herman is. Some things you just can't tell him at all.

(*Albert looks to Robert, who takes a deep breath and starts again.*)

ROBERT: Mrs. Lawrence, I know you're his wife . . . a-and it's not that I'm trying to keep anything from you. But this is something your husband needs to decide to share with you. I don't have any trouble with your being there with him when we talk about his condition—so long as that's what Herman would like. What I'm wanting to do now, though, is just let you know that your husband has a condition that is going to need serious attention and, given what my father's told me about the way your husband responds to news about his health, I just want to make sure that any discussion we have with him doesn't wind up doing more harm than good. (*Realizing that he has somewhat misspoken, Robert quickly starts again.*) What I mean is that I think this is your husband's decision, but given his tendency to . . . overreact to situations that have to do with his health, I want to be able to present him with information in a way that doesn't . . . well, let's just say that isn't counterproductive. Do you understand what I mean?

LINDA: (*looking to Albert and then back to Robert*) I understand what you're saying. But if you're planning on telling my husband that there's something seriously wrong with him and then expecting him to make a decision about what to do . . . it just doesn't work that way with Herman. I don't know what's the matter yet, but I can tell you now that if it's serious, then by telling Herman the only thing you're going to get out of it is withdrawal. Herman will close up like a clam. He'll say it's not true. He'll deny it. He might even get up and walk right out.

ROBERT: Isn't there some way to talk to him about these things? There must be *some* level on which he can discuss his health.

(*Linda looks perplexed, as if she's dealing with a slow child. Again she looks to Albert, who this time just shrugs his shoulders.*)

ROBERT: (*Genuinely bemused, Robert looks to both his father and Linda.*) What do either of you do when he has an infection and needs to take antibiotics?

ALBERT: In the last few years we just tell him these pills will make him better, and not to worry about it.

(*As Robert ponders this response both Linda and Albert wait. Linda has recognized that at least for the moment Robert is in charge, and so she tries to be patient.*)

ROBERT: How do you think Herman would react if he was told that his abdominal condition needed further treatment, and then I asked him whether he'd like us—you, me, and my father, that is—to simply arrange what needed doing?

LINDA: Um . . .

ROBERT: One of my concerns here is that Herman be given the chance to take part in the decision-making regarding his health care. (*a little defensively*) I'm not trying to call into question you and my father's experience dealing with Herman. But your husband is a competent person who deserves to be treated with the same respect we give to others. If your husband says that he would feel more comfortable having you, or you and my father and I, making his health care decisions for him, then so be it. But if he wants to be more involved, it seems to me that we have to respect his decision, even though it might not be the one we would make. (*Robert pauses*) Does that make sense?

LINDA: (*a little defiantly now*) It makes sense. But not for Herman. Herman will go to pieces. He might not do it right here at your office, but within a couple three days he won't be able to deal with it at all. He'll either act like it doesn't exist and refuse to do anything about it or he'll get to thinking that there's no hope and therefore no point in doing anything about whatever it is that's going on.

ROBERT: It's not at all that I don't believe you, Mrs. Lawrence. But I'm trying to discern whether there isn't some way of including your husband in the decision-making process without precipitating the kind of reaction you've come to know. Is it possible that it's fear that makes him react like that?

LINDA: Of course it's fear. My husband's not an idiot. But this is a fear that started in childhood for him. In any case, it's certainly not something he's going to get over because you have some new idea about how he ought to react.

(*Linda is now starting to react a bit herself. She is already worried about her husband's condition and is now starting to get visibly exasperated. Robert perceives this and attempts to recoup the situation. He gives Linda a moment to settle down and then responds.*)

ROBERT: I think, Mrs. Lawrence, that we *can* resolve this in a way that we both find acceptable, but we're going to have to work on it . . . together. (*Robert pauses, then begins to push himself away from his desk.*) Say, um . . . would you like something to drink? I was thinking of getting something for myself.

LINDA: Um, sure. Uh, anything diet would be fine.

ROBERT: You, Dad?

ALBERT: Actually, why don't you let me get it. You want a Coke, right?

ROBERT: Mm-hm. Thanks. (*Robert turns to Linda as Albert leaves the room to get them drinks. There is an awkward silence, then Robert begins.*) So . . . been a pretty long day here. How 'bout you?

LINDA: Yeah, I guess it has. (*trying to make small talk until Albert comes back*) We've got a set of grandkids coming over on Friday. They always expect me to have baked something. I don't like to disappoint them, so I spent most of this morning shopping.

(*Albert returns with a diet soda for Linda, a Coke for Robert, and iced tea for himself.*)

ROBERT: (*looking interested and trying to make their interaction more "conversational"*) So, what are you going to bake?

LINDA: Oh, the usual—chocolate chip cookies, some banana bread, enough for them to take some home. Our daughter's so busy, she doesn't have time for much baking.

ALBERT: (*chiding his son a little*) If you're nice to her, she'll probably bring you in some. It's worth it, let me tell you. They're good! (*Linda smiles a smile of genuine affection.*)

LINDA: Oh, Dr. Bang. You always know how to flatter me.

(*The mood is pleasant. But as Linda remembers the nature of her visit to Dr. Bang, an awkward silence develops. Finally, Robert takes a deep breath and starts.*)

ROBERT: Mrs. Lawrence . . . what I'd like to do is run a few ideas by you and (*sensing that Linda is starting to react again, Robert holds up his hands as if to brace her*) . . . and just get your reactions. We're not deciding anything yet. (*slowing and softening his voice*) I'm just trying to get a sense of how (*again, Robert holds up his hands*) *without disconcerting your husband* we can give him the opportunity to participate *if he wants.*

(*Robert looks Linda in the eye and waits. Linda takes a deep breath and readies herself to listen. On her face is a look that says: "I'll listen but it's not going to work."*)

ROBERT: Let's say the two of you came in tomorrow or the next day and I explained to Herman that we got some results back from the tests we ran to figure out what's causing his abdominal pain. What would he do then? Would he ask what the test results said?

LINDA: Probably not. He'd probably just sit there and wait. Like I told you, Herman tries to avoid dealing with his health problems.

ROBERT: OK. Just so I know. But just for the sake of argument, let's say he did ask. If I continued by saying something like, "Well, Herman, it looks like your abdominal pain is more involved than we thought and there's some further treatment that needs to be done," what do you think he'd say?

LINDA: I'm tellin' ya. He'd probably just sit there.

ROBERT: OK, alright. So now imagine I then went on to say that there are a number of ways to proceed, but that we need to know what he wants. If he wants to, he can delegate his decision-making to you. That is, he could decide that, as his wife, he wanted *you* to be responsible for finding out about his condition and deciding what should be done. He could even decide that he wanted *you* to be the one to tell him what was going on and what needed doing. How do you think he'd react to that?

LINDA: That's how it works already.

ROBERT: I understand that. I'm just trying to get a fuller understanding of how Herman would react if he was given that option.

LINDA: (*Not understanding the point of this inquiry, Linda turns to Albert and with an imploring look asks what is not really a question.*) Dr. Bang, you know Herman. You know that I always make these kind of decisions for him.

ALBERT: I think Robert understands that Linda. He just wants to know what Herman would say if he was actually presented with the option. That is, would Herman *say* that he wants you to make his decisions for him or would he say that *he* wants to make them?

LINDA: Well, I don't really know, Dr. Bang. It's just something we've worked out over the years. We've never talked about it specifically.

ROBERT: (*gently, but also prodding*) Mrs. Lawrence, how would *you* feel about giving him that option?

LINDA: I . . . I don't know.

ROBERT: (*again, gently prodding*) Are you unsure because you don't know what he'd choose to do?

LINDA: I . . . I guess that's it. I've never really thought about it before. (*Linda takes a moment to think about it, then continues.*) I'd be pretty scared, though, if he said he did want to know. I wouldn't think he knew what he was doing.

ROBERT: How do you think you'd handle it if he did?

LINDA: Did what?

ROBERT: If he said he did want to know.

LINDA: I don't know . . . I'd probably tell him he didn't want to know.

ROBERT: Well, could you imagine him being concerned enough *to* want to know? I guess I'm asking whether you could accept him wanting to know—and I understand that this is not something he's dealt with well in the past. But do you think you could accept his decision to want to be informed, and maybe even take part in deciding what should be done? I realize it'd be a major change, but . . .

LINDA: Doctor, it . . . it's hard to put into words because . . . well, it's not like Herman can't make decisions. But when it comes to his health he just gets to thinking that it's beyond his control, and so long as he doesn't know about it . . . how should I put it . . . (*Linda searches for words*) I guess, he figures that fate can't get to him so long as he doesn't know. So he tries not to know.

ROBERT: (*very sympathetically*) That must be really hard for you. It puts a lot of responsibility on you.

LINDA: I guess it does. But Herman's such a good man, I just hate to see him suffer with it. (*Linda pauses and then continues.*) Where he grew up in Pittsburgh, he says that during the depression neighbors and cousins seemed to be dying all the time from TB and pneumonia and, well, I guess they were poor and there was lots of disease . . . (*Linda shakes her head as she talks.*) And coming out here to San Francisco was like an escape from all that death. And then when so much of his family started to die, it was like he just couldn't escape it. So instead he shut it out. (*Linda falls quiet.*)

ROBERT: I guess we all do that in one way or another. (*Robert waits a few moments and then continues.*) The question is whether we can help Herman deal with his situation in a way that doesn't threaten him. You've worked real hard to protect him from that, but now he's at a point that, I think we need to find another way to keep him from feeling threatened. Anyone who used to weld hundreds of feet up in the air is certainly someone with a lot of courage. What I'm hoping that we can do is find a way to bring that out. Obviously, we want to do that carefully, to minimize the risk that he'll decompensate. But we all might be surprised at what he's capable of.

LINDA: I'd like to think you're right. But I just don't know—it could devastate him. (*Linda turns to Albert, searches his eyes for some reassurance, and then asks*) Dr. Bang, what do you think? You know how Herman is.

(*Albert takes a moment in answering. He looks toward Robert briefly, as if to remind him of their agreement, and then looks back to Linda.*)

ALBERT: Initially . . . I tend to share your skepticism and I worry that Herman will react badly. Herman is a good man, but we both know that he's not very good at this sort of thing. On the other hand, I think my son's correct. Herman is a grown man and deserves to have a say in how his life goes. And if we're going to respect that, then we have to respect it, even when we're not sure what he'll say. Believe me, I understand that for you this is very scary. There's no guarantee that Herman will be able to deal with this, at least not well. But if we're careful and pay attention I think we can minimize the risk that he'll decompensate psychologically. In other words, I think we should give him a chance—with the understanding that we'll have to be careful and that in spite of our best efforts we might fail . . . (*Albert continues, his tone a little more serious now*) *Your husband is going to need treatment*—and in the long run he's probably going to learn what's going on, anyway. If we work with him now we at least give him the opportunity to overcome his fears. I think we have to have some faith that he can do it.

(*Looking defeated, Linda nods silently. She literally dreads the prospect of being with her husband when Dr. Bang tries to talk to him. She remembers Herman's anxiety and out-and-out fear when he had that skin wart thing removed, and how difficult it had been for her husband when they visited Herman's little brother in the hospital last year just before he died. Linda is a little wary of the younger Dr. Bang. But she trusts "her" Dr. Bang and she agrees to come in with Herman in a couple of days. When she gets home, she doesn't tell her husband that she's been to see Dr. Bang.*

When Linda and Herman come in on Thursday afternoon about 3:30 one can see that Linda is working very hard not to be nervous. Herman sees that his wife is a bit distracted but figures it is just one of her moods that probably has to do with their grandchildren coming to visit the next day. They are seated in Robert's office on the far side of the room in two chairs angled toward the desk. There is another chair just across from them also angled toward the desk. As they wait Herman talks about taking his grandchildren out to the zoo when they come. The zoo is at the end of the bus line, and it always seems so peaceful, like a refuge from the rest of the city. Just then, Robert walks in followed by his father. Herman stands up to greet them while Linda remains seated.)

ROBERT: Hello Mr. Lawrence, it's good to see you again.

HERMAN: You, too. (*The two men shake hands. As Robert then nods to Linda and moves around the desk to sit behind it, Herman and Albert greet each other warmly.*)

ALBERT: Well, hello Herman!

HERMAN: Hello Dr. Bang! (*A much larger man than Albert, Herman clasps Albert's smaller hand with his two big palms as they shake.*)

ALBERT: (*warmly*) So, how've you been, Herman? I haven't seen you in a while.

HERMAN: (*also with genuine affection*) Mm, not so bad. How about yourself?

ALBERT: Pretty good. Staying healthy, working hard.

HERMAN: (*gesturing toward Robert*) And you've got your son here with you now. You did a good job. He's going to make a fine doctor.

ALBERT: (*joking*) Well, he's got a great role model, you know. (*The two men chuckle as Robert shakes his head and Linda waits anxiously. They then sit down and Herman speaks, now more businesslike.*)

HERMAN: You know, Dr. Bang, if this is about the pain in my stomach . . . it's really not bothering me that much. I wouldn't have even come in if it wasn't for Linda, here. She's always worrying that I don't pay enough attention to my health.

ALBERT: Well, I'll tell you what, Herman. Since Robert, here, has been taking care of you this time around, I'll let him do the talking. You know, he's going to take over the whole practice in a few years so me and Lienne can enjoy our retirement in peace.

HERMAN: Ah, retirement is a good thing. (*Herman turns to Robert, who is leaning forward a bit with his forearms resting on the desk, his fingers interlaced.*) So . . . ?

ROBERT: Well, I'm pleased to say that the majority of your tests were entirely normal. In many ways you're a very healthy person and except for enjoying your wife's cooking a little too much, maybe (*Robert wags a finger at Herman's belly*), you're doing a good job keeping yourself out of trouble. (*Robert pauses and notices Linda's fearful look.*) I am glad to hear you say that your abdomen isn't bothering you that much. But one of the things those tests we ran told us is that antacids aren't going to do the trick. (*Robert watches Herman's face for any sign of anxiety. Herman looks almost stoic and so Robert continues.*) What I'm saying is that you're going to need a different kind of treatment and we wanted to talk with you about that. (*Robert looks inquiringly at Herman, who says nothing.*) There are a number of ways we can go about this. My father tells me that your wife usually takes care of this end of things for you. If you want, we can keep on doing it that way. If you've got things you need to do, we can keep your wife informed and you can just find out what you need to from her. (*Robert pauses and looks to Herman, waiting.*) Is that how you'd like us to work this? Or . . . well, what would you like?

HERMAN: Well . . . I guess that depends. I'm supposed to go on a trip up to Seattle next month to visit my son and his family. They rented a cabin out on Vancouver Island and we're supposed to spend about ten days there. Is this treatment you're talking about going to interfere with that?

ROBERT: Well, maybe. Depending on how soon we start and when in August you're planning on leaving . . .

HERMAN: We're supposed to be up there by the twenty-second.

ROBERT: Hm . . . let's see, that's a full six weeks from now. That certainly gives us a chance to get you taken care of and back up to speed. You might still be a little tired toward the end of the day. But if everything goes as we hope, you should be able to go walking through the woods up there without too much trouble. (*Robert sees Albert quietly nodding his head, letting him know that this is a good pace. Robert waits for a response.*)

HERMAN: That's good. I've been looking forward to this trip all summer.

ROBERT: At this point I don't see any problem. There'll be some things we'll want to do when you get back in the fall to follow up and make sure that everything's taken care of. But barring something unexpected you should be in good shape . . . um . . . I guess the question I have for you is . . . uh . . . how you'd like to uh . . . decide how to proceed here. Would you like us to just discuss it with your wife and have her get back to you or would you like to be more centrally involved? (*Linda appears to cringe at this as Robert braces himself for whatever will happen.*)

HERMAN: Is it an ulcer? My son had one of those.

ROBERT: (*a little apprehensively*) No.

HERMAN: And it's not gonna mean I have to cut out spicy food is it?

ROBERT: I wouldn't think so.

(*Despite being a little perplexed and obviously curious, Herman seems to have been put at ease by Robert—at least so far. By contrast, Linda wears a tight smile that makes Albert think back to the new recruits he used to see in the service when they would line up for their first parachute jump. And yet, when Herman looks to Linda for reassurance, it is there.*)

HERMAN: Hmph. Well, I guess it all sounds fine.

ROBERT: (*a little confused*) What does?

HERMAN: That you can treat me without me having to scrub my trip.

ROBERT: Oh, right. So . . . um, would you like to know more about your condition or would you rather have your wife handle it?

HERMAN: (*not seeming to understand what Robert's trying to get at*) She's right here. You can go on ahead.

ROBERT: What I mean is, do you want to know what we think you're going to need to do and why?

HERMAN: Uh . . . I guess so.

ROBERT: The reason I ask is that some people don't like to know, and if you're one of those people, that's OK. But you need to decide.

HERMAN: (*finally getting it, and now a little more circumspect*) I get it. You want to know whether I want to know.

ROBERT: (*nodding his head*) Right.

HERMAN: Is this something that's going to upset me? (*looking over toward Albert and then back to Robert*) I don't always deal with health problems real well.

ROBERT: Well, you do have a problem. But it's the kind of problem that we can do something about. (*Herman furrows his brow as Robert pauses, then continues.*) I've been told that health problems make you . . . well, a little nervous.

HERMAN: (*starting to get nervous*) More than nervous. They . . . they unhinge me.

ROBERT: (*as soothingly as he can*) I understand that. That's why I'm saying right up front that what's going on with you is something we know how to deal with. We have a lot of experience with it and . . . mmh, it's not something to get *real* worried about. We can deal with it and we will. The question is whether you want to be a part of that or whether you want us (*Robert makes a sweeping gesture that takes in Linda and Albert and himself*) to handle it all for you. That's what I need to know.

HERMAN: (*abruptly, and catching everyone off guard*) Do I have cancer? (*With this, Linda shuts her eyes, as if in despair.*)

ROBERT: Uh . . . that depends what you mean.

HERMAN: I don't follow you. Either I have it or I don't, right?

ROBERT: Mm, depends. You see . . . well, imagine I asked you whether someone was a welder. Chances are you'd say that depends. It depends on what you *mean* by welding. Strictly speaking, someone who makes computer chips down in Silicon Valley is as much a welder as someone who's working one hundred feet in the air on a steel beam, right? But if I'm an insurance agent trying to figure out what that person's premium should be, there's a world of difference in terms of what "being a welder" means. (*Herman nods.*) The only thing that "cancer" means is that of the trillions and trillions of cells in your body *some of them* are growing irregularly. Some people who don't know any better think that having cancer means you're going to die from it or may be disfigured or be in horrible pain for the rest of your life. Now, if *that's* what *you* mean by cancer, then I'd say that that's not the case.

HERMAN: (*Herman avoids Robert's gaze and as he fixes his eyes on Robert's hands, which are still resting on the desk, Herman's voice is grave.*) Everyone who *I've* known who had cancer died. (*Herman's voice trails off.*)

ROBERT: I can show you people who twenty years ago had what you have now and are doing fine. They go camping up on Vancouver Island every year. Ask my father, he'll tell you about people just like you—your age, your health, your condition—who are healthy and enjoying life. (*Robert gestures toward Albert and, reluctantly, Herman looks up.*)

ALBERT: He's right, Herman. I've had lots of patients just like you who are now the picture of health. Robert, why don't you draw a picture of the large bowel and I'll explain to Herman what needs to be done. OK?

(*Robert gets out an 11 × 14 legal pad and quickly sketches the contents of a normal abdomen. As Robert does this, Linda reaches over and takes Herman's hand. Linda looks to reassure Herman that everything will be alright, but despite this Herman has the appearance of a man who is ready to give up. Robert finishes his sketch and, leaning forward across the desk, turns it around so that Herman and Linda can see. Albert scoots forward and using the drawing begins to explain as Herman and Linda look on.*)

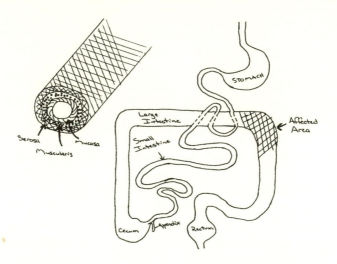

ALBERT: You see, Herman, you, and everyone else for that matter, have an enormous amount of intestine—about twenty-five feet or so in all. The small intestine here (*Albert points to the drawing*) begins at the lower part of your stomach and goes around and around until it ends right here (*he points again*) at the bottom of the cecum. And if my son had been a little more diligent (*Albert says wryly*), he would have put the appendix right here, where the cecum is. (*Albert draws in an appendix.*) From the cecum onward is your large intestine. It has an ascending part (*Albert traces it as he speaks*), a transverse part, and a descending part. And then, of course, you have the rectum and the anus. Now of this whole twenty-five feet worth of intestines, you've got a problem right here. (*Albert shades in the top third of the descending colon including the flexure where it joins with*

the transverse colon.) That's about nine inches. (*Albert pauses and makes sure that Herman catches his emphasis.*) *Nine inches out of twenty-five feet.* Now the colon is sort of like a garden hose, but with three kinds of layers. (*Albert draws an oblique view of a hollow cylinder with three layers that he then labels.*) The inner layer is called the mucosa. It's the one in direct contact with food as it passes through the intestine. The middle layer is called the muscularis, because it's made up of muscles. The outer layer is called the serosa. Are you following me here?

HERMAN: Yessir. (*Linda nods. Both Herman and Linda are captivated.*)

ALBERT: Well, colon cancer—that is, irregularly growing cells in the colon—almost always begin in the mucosa, the innermost layer. Those irregularly growing cells usually form a ring in that layer. When they've formed *that* ring, these irregular cells then grow into the muscularis. When they've formed a ring in that layer they then go on to grow in the outermost layer, the serosa. At that stage of the game, these irregular cells can work their way into other parts of your body. It's usually the case that these cells begin to invade structures that lie close by. But once these irregular cells get beyond the serosa, here (*Albert points*), they can also get into your lymphatic system or your blood, both of which go all over your body. That's how these irregular cells spread to places like your liver and your lungs and your bones and so forth. Now, what's wrong with these cells is that they don't know when to stop growing, and that's why we need to take them out wherever we find them. Are you with me, still?

HERMAN: Uh-huh. (*Linda nods.*)

ALBERT: OK. Now if these cells are just in one spot it makes the job of removing them lots easier. We just send you to surgery and they take out that part. Just like when they take out your appendix. In *your* case, that means taking out about nine or ten inches of your descending colon, right here. (*Again, Albert points.*) That's *nine or ten inches* out of a total of *twenty-five feet* of intestine. The reason we can do that with you is that your irregular cells haven't gotten out of the middle layer. They're still in the muscularis. They haven't made it to the outside layer or into the adjoining parts of your body. Now when the surgeons are in there, they'll probably take out various lymph nodes to make sure that these cells haven't gotten into your lymph system, which they shouldn't have at this point. And as follow-up we may want to give you some medicine that will kill any irregular cells that by chance got out early. Of course, we can't be certain that none of these cells *have* gotten out already. But if we move on this quickly we can remove those nine or ten inches of your colon before it becomes more likely that those irregular cells will get out.

(*Albert looks to Herman and Linda, who both seem a little dazed. Robert nods to Albert, indicating that they seem to have understood what Albert has been explaining.*)

ALBERT: Does that make sense to you so far? (*Albert looks at Herman and Linda, who both nod.*) As you can see, you're in real good shape here. We're talking about *less than a foot* out of twenty-five feet of intestine and, as far as we know, no spread of these irregular cells beyond those few inches. What you have to understand, though, is that the reason we're in good shape is because it's early in the game. The longer we wait the worse it gets. If you're going to take advantage of your position, we'll need to act quickly. You ought to be in surgery by next week. Are you clear on all that? (*Linda looks at Herman supportively as Herman looks first to Robert and then back at Albert.*) What you've got appears to be very localized and by acting quickly the chances are *overwhelming* that it is curable.

HERMAN: (*despairingly*) So I *do* have cancer.

LINDA: *Herman,* you heard what the doctor said, there are different kinds of cancer. And the kind you have isn't what you're thinking.

HERMAN: (*despairingly*) But I *do* have cancer.

ALBERT: I know it doesn't seem this way, but you're a very fortunate man, Herman. You've been worried for the last fifteen to twenty years that you were in danger. A lot of people in your family had problems with their health and . . .

HERMAN: And all of them died.

ALBERT: What I'm saying, Herman, is that you don't have to worry anymore that you're like the rest of your family. You're in a position to fight this *and win*. You can get this treated. You've already outlived everyone in your family. Now it's just a matter of using your advantage to avoid their fate . . . because it doesn't have to be *your* fate. (*Albert pauses and watches Herman for a moment, who seems almost stunned into silence.*) I know this is hard for you, Herman. It would be hard for anybody. But the only way to beat this, and you can, is by facing up to it. This is important, Herman. It's as important as what you did on the Golden Gate Bridge. (*At this, Herman looks up. The situation seems to register more fully in his eyes.*) Are there things that either of you have questions about? (*Herman sits there in silence. Finally, Linda speaks.*)

LINDA: H-how would we arrange this?

ALBERT: We can take care of all of that. I've already spoken with a good friend of mine, Dr. Lo, who does these operations all the time, and he could work you into his schedule the middle of next week. We'd need to know by tomorrow, though.

LINDA: (*looking at Herman, who is sitting there almost helplessly, and then back to Albert*) I understand. Are there things we need to do?

ALBERT: Well, you need to make sure that you understand what treatment involves and agree to consent to it, including the various risks. Herman would need to go into the hospital on Monday and be there for a few days to run tests and to get him ready for his surgery. But other than that, not much else.

(*Albert looks sympathetically at Herman, whose eyes are fixed on the floor. Albert then looks back to Linda, who he knows will have a very long weekend ahead of her. Almost reading Albert's mind, Linda comments*)

LINDA: Our grandkids are coming this weekend.

ALBERT: I think that'll be good for the two of you. Maybe it'll take your mind off this a bit. Kids remind you that almost anything is possible. Isn't that right, Herman?

HERMAN: (*looking up from the floor, still somewhat dazed*) Huh?

LINDA: (*doing her best to smile*) Dr. Bang said that it was a good thing the kids are coming this weekend. You can take them out to the zoo and show them your favorite places again.

HERMAN: Yeah, I guess so.

ROBERT: Herman, is there anything you want to ask? Anything at all.

HERMAN: (*there is a long pause, then*) Uh . . . I don't think so.

ROBERT: You, Linda?

LINDA: I think we're going to need to go home and talk about this. We'll get back to you tomorrow, if that's alright. (*Linda's tone reminds Robert of a cleaning woman he knew from his residency, overworked and unempowered, but defiant just the same. Robert's face expresses sympathy, but inside he's much more unsure of his feelings.*)

ALBERT: If there's anything you need, just give me a call—even if it's just to talk. You have my home phone number. This is important, and I know it's not easy. Herman? (*Herman, who has been staring off blankly, looks at Albert.*) Herman, you have a lot of power here. But if it's going to be used effectively, you have to exercise it. You need to follow through with this. Talk with Linda about it tonight and I'll expect to hear back from you tomorrow. We can deal with this. But we need to act quickly and we're going to need your help so that we can make sure you get up to Vancouver Island on time. Alright?

(*Albert stands and the others follow suit. Herman shakes Robert's hand and then Albert's. Linda nods politely to Robert and, as she leads her husband from the office, quietly says to Albert, "I'll give you a call." Albert and Robert watch as Linda puts her arm around her husband's waist and goes out the door of the office. Robert and his father stand quietly until Herman and Linda are gone.)*

ROBERT: (*looking over at his father*) So? What do you think?

ALBERT: I don't know. I hope we did the right thing. I guess we'll find out tomorrow.

⑥ Appreciating Autonomy

Clearly, respecting patients' autonomy can be a complex task, made all the more difficult when one has to make judgments about their values *for them*. But there are also special difficulties associated with patients' own judgments about their values, particularly when those judgments involve greatly imprudent decisions. One looming issue is whether it is possible to rationally make greatly imprudent decisions, decisions that for want of foresight and wisdom do not show sound practical judgment. Clearly, to be prudent Sally need not always do what is in her best interest, only not do what is in her worst or significantly bad interest. Roughly, an imprudent act is one that involves self-sacrifice without good countervailing reasons. Though we commonly recognize that imprudence takes stronger and weaker forms, often we forget that at base imprudence is a *normative* concept. Many decisions once thought imprudent are no longer so, and so too the reverse. Hence we must beware of regarding certain decisions or kinds of decisions as de jure imprudent. We also must beware of assuming that prudence comes only from objective reasoning and logical analysis. For society's assessments of imprudence are as often based on accepted bias as they are on accepted knowledge—and what it means to live in the present is that often we cannot distinguish between the two. In fact, part of what we have learned from modern critiques of science and rationality is that no clear criteria establish what should and should not count as "rational."[1] This is not to say that the terms *imprudent* and *rational* have no appropriate use. Since we have no choice but to dwell in the present, our assessments must be based on our current understanding of the world. Nonetheless, when we ask, "Is it possible to rationally make greatly imprudent decisions?" our response should be sufficiently flexible to accommodate the (necessarily) nonobjective nature of both the terms *imprudent* and *rational*.

Is great imprudence consistent with rationality? When dealing with autonomous human beings, the answer depends on whether the charge of imprudence is based on the standards and values of the agent or those of society. Clearly, people will disagree over what level of risk is acceptable and how much benefit is derived from a particular outcome. Take, for example, Sally's decision to experiment with LSD or hitchhike alone across the United States or smoke cigarettes. Friends and family may judge Sally's decision as greatly imprudent according to *their* standards. They may be convinced that there are better, less risky ways to achieve the experience or adventure sought in such activities. But do such external assessments tell against the rationality of Sally's decision? I think not. So long as Sally meets the rationality requirement of autonomy and her decision is consistent with her own standards and values, it is no sign of nonrationality that her decision deviates from social norms. The normative aspect of rationality is already accounted for by Sally's qualifying as autonomous. Demanding greater adherence to social norms has nothing to do with rationality but rather with foisting preferences and priorities on others. It is often both mistaken and arrogant to believe that our particular assessments of value and worth are shared by others or, worse yet, that they should be. Thus, when "great imprudence" is understood as an *external* assessment it can be consistent with rationality.

It is quite another matter, however, when the charge is that Sally's decision is greatly imprudent according to *her own* standards and values. When Sally's decision does not show sound practical judgment because it is internally inconsistent, this *does* defeat the procedural aspect of rationality. It simply is not consistent with rationality to act contrary to all one's values and standards. Thus, when "great imprudence" is an internal assessment it cannot be consistent with rationality. Of course, what counts as "greatly imprudent according to *one's own* standards and values" is not always a straightforward matter. Not all of our values and standards are entirely consistent with one another, and many of them are context dependent. Moreover, our values and standards change, and so uncharacteristic behavior, even when it is potentially very harmful, by itself does no more than raise a red flag, prompting us to further inquiry. There are many perfectly rational reasons to act in uncharacteristic ways that bring one harm.[2] Additionally, one may have very different priorities concerning one's future selves. Since "connectedness is nearly always weaker over longer periods," Sally can rationally care less about her distant future than about her present.[3] To pass judgment on the nature of a decision, we must attend to the (mysterious) process of decision-making and the influences involved.

So whether great imprudence is consistent with rationality depends on how imprudence is defined. If imprudence is defined in terms of the standards and values of others, then great imprudence *is* consistent with rationality, but if imprudence is defined in terms of the standards and values of the agent herself, then it *is not*. In assessing the imprudence of Sally's decisions, however, we should beware of attempts to oversimplify what counts as Sally's standards and values. All too often people overlook the fullness of Sally's desires, drives, intentions, plans, convictions, and principles. Instead, they equate prudence with an oversimplified version of "in her best interests," a version that is then hard-pressed to accommodate autonomous decisions that depart from previous modes of behavior or priorities. Occasionally, one must look hard and deep to determine whether an apparently imprudent decision is consistent with Sally's own standards and values. But if it is consistent, I will argue that we must respect Sally's prerogative to make it.

The Value of Autonomy

Throughout this discussion, I have claimed that being considered autonomous is a fundamental and an intrinsic value.[4] Moreover, I have suggested that there are compelling reasons to respect patients' autonomous PSR decisions. What arguments exist to support such assertions?

Clearly, autonomy is not necessary to qualify as a person, per se. No reasonable individual believes that a five year old or someone with Down's syndrome is any less a "person" for their lacking autonomy. No reasonable individual holds that nonautonomous human beings can be used merely as the means to another person's end or should be loved or cared for any less. Indeed, these people often receive the most attention precisely because they lack the ability to govern themselves. But despite the regard accorded such individuals, those who lack autonomy do not qualify for the same regard we ascribe to autonomous beings. There are important differences between individuals who possess and exercise autonomy and those who do not. Autonomy guarantees one a place within society, both in terms of opportunity and responsibility. For in large part what allows us to hold people morally accountable, to tie moral value or significance to their actions, to respect their goals, to give credence to their conceptions of the good life, to see them as full, active members of human society is their ability to be self-governing, to think and act autonomously. Similarly, with regard to ourselves, to have dignity and self-esteem, much less integrity,[5] one must possess the self-monitoring and self-critical capacities constituent of autonomy. It is precisely because I can develop and reason through and criticize my own beliefs and values and priorities that we (including myself) are prepared to heap praise and blame and responsibility on *me* for their content.[6]

In point of fact, it is not clear what conception of human society would be left without autonomy. Could our conception of justice survive? or democracy? or moral or intellectual judgment? or even education? Without the assumption that people have the capacity to be self-governing it is unclear how the personal or institutional expectations that form the basis for the functioning of society can even get off the ground. Certainly, to take seriously others' aspirations and values and ideas, much less think them worthy of our respect, we must suppose those aspirations and values and ideas arise from a person who possesses standards of self-critical evaluation. If Sally is incapable of critically evaluating her situation and formulating, revising, and pursuing her ends or goals in an intelligible manner, then she is no more than a mouthpiece that emits words. What reason is there to consider Sally's pronouncements representative of her moral being unless she has the capacity to assess and endorse them? Without that kind of consideration, we cannot treat her as equal. Indeed, if we are to regard Sally as genuinely, fully one of us, as a moral equal, as a prerequisite she must qualify as an author of changes in the world and not merely as a stenographer. In sum, autonomy is a necessary condition for conceiving of others as (our) moral equals, and hence is intrinsically valuable.

Why it is necessary to view individuals as the author of their scripts to regard them with the respect and consideration due an equal, full participating member of human society is a separate question. One possible answer is that the value we impute to autonomous activity is genuinely a "basic value," without a source, that must stand or fall on its own merits.[7] An interesting empirical study would be to assess the universality of wanting to make a mark in the world, "not in order that it might be made, but in order to have made it."[8] If such a drive for authorship was found in all cultures, it would strengthen the argument for the central importance of autonomy as a value. Irrespective of such a finding, however, I think it is clear that we do regard autonomy as a prerequisite to being considered a full, equal member of society.

The question that remains is whether the fundamental value we place on autonomy drives us (in all cases) to respect patients' autonomous PSR decisions. Clearly, there are many perfectly good reasons to override autonomous decisions, per se, including protection of others from harm and concerns for justice. But what about PSR decisions? I argued earlier that unless we regard certain matters as PSR it is hard to conceive of individuals as truly self-governing. PSR decisions are defined in part precisely by their exemption from other-regarding concerns. Hence, if there are good reasons to override PSR decisions, those reasons cannot be based on the interests of others. Additionally, I already have argued that if one is acting *out of respect for* a patient's autonomy it is not possible to at the same time be overriding her *present* exercise of autonomy.[9] So what rationales for overriding PSR decisions remain? As I understand it, there are three: promoting the patient's future capacity for autonomy, promoting the patient's future exercise of autonomy, and promoting the patient's well-being.

The problem with the first two options is that their value is unclear. Since acting *out of respect for* autonomy entails respecting the *present* exercise of autonomy, both of these rationales for overriding PSR decisions must have as their goal some unrealized future state or event.

Now this is not incomprehensible, but it does seem strange at best to value a future state over its present realization. As John Dewey explains, under such a value scheme "when the future arrives it is only after all another despised present."[10] Surely it will be no more important to respect the exercise of autonomy at some future date, unless what one is meaning to promote/respect is not autonomy at all. And that is just the point, that so long as one is meaning to act *out of respect for* autonomy, as opposed to something else, there can be no other meaningful focus beyond the present exercise of autonomy. Certainly it is conceivable to locate the value of autonomy in some future exercise or state of being, but it would have to *remain* an unrealized future state or exercise. It is simply unclear how one can attach meaning to "being autonomous" if autonomy's value resides in a permanently unrealized form.

If my arguments are right, I suspect that I have merely forced many would-be paternalists to change the justification for their interventions. I have forced them to acknowledge that their paternalistic intention to override patients' present autonomous PSR decisions cannot be grounded in respect for autonomy, but instead must be justified in terms of promoting well-being. But if this is all I have accomplished, I am quite satisfied. For if I have denied paternalists this justification, I have denied them access to one of the strongest and most meaningful moral principles our society has to offer. And if my arguments regarding PSR decisions are right, then paternalists' failure to respect patients' autonomous PSR decisions is nothing less than a failure to treat patients as moral equals.

Of course criticism against paternalistic interventions to override patients' present autonomous PSR decisions does not end here, for the paternalistic arguments from well-being are themselves open to a number of telling objections. John Stuart Mill, for example, defended the importance of an individual's self-determination on at least three separate utilitarian grounds. First, holding that autonomy is constituent of humans' highest good and that "the mental and moral, like the muscular powers, are improved only by being used,"[11] Mill argued that *in order* to realize human happiness, the capacity for autonomy must be promoted and its exercise respected. Mill also argued that in the vast majority of cases it will be more conducive to overall happiness to allow individuals to be self-determining, rather than for others to make decisions for them. And finally, Mill also echoed Thoreau's skepticism about the intentions of those who would intervene to do us good. Clearly, Mill's points cannot be demonstrated as necessary conditions. But Mill does provide strong arguments that individuals are virtually always better equipped to know their own best interests, that often the real motivations for interfering with the exercise of someone's autonomy have to do more with the desire to control or to shape others like oneself, and that the very exercise of autonomy produces a significant degree of satisfaction and, therefore, utility.

An alternate response to would-be paternalists is simply that it is wrong to regard well-being as more important than self-governance.[12] In the first place, both our intuition and our general tendency is to value self-made decisions, even when such a course begets mistakes. It is more than just a philosophical cliché that it is better to be Socrates dissatisfied than a pig satisfied. We think being controlled is terribly wrong irrespective of the advantages of such control. We find it intrinsically valuable to exercise our autonomy. Second, and perhaps more powerfully, overriding the exercise of autonomy to promote that individual's own well-being is wrong because that individual is being used merely as a means to an end. We think it wrong to tie down an autonomous patient against her will simply to benefit HCPs, though every day thousands of elderly patients in nursing homes are physically restrained simply to ease the burden of care-giving. But what makes such an act any more appropriate merely because the benefit goes to the patient? In the absence of consent, overriding the wishes of an autonomous patient to promote her well-being transforms her into a mere instrumentality, which sets up a contradiction at the least. For it is the basis of our moral system to treat other autonomous beings as moral equals and not simply as a means to an end, and to treat autonomous patients as moral equals is to respect their right to make PSR decisions.

Before going on, let me say a few words about the notion of rights and why until now I have tried to avoid using the term, instead substituting words such as *prerogative*. In recent years rights-based theories have come under increasing scrutiny for their reliance on a nonrelational conception of human society. A particular danger with rights talk lies in its apparent endorsement of an atomistic conception of individuals that neglects the social nature of human existence and fails to attend to those aspects of human relationships that sustain human society. For this reason I have avoided it. And yet speaking of rights is useful, for rights convey a definiteness often important for talking about assignments of power. In particular, rights indicate who gets to have final say about a matter, and frequently rights also designate correlative responsibilities. I believe that safeguarding patients' exercise of autonomy in PSR matters is sufficiently important that it warrants speaking in terms of rights, and that is why I have switched terminology. Moreover, the present context suggests a reasonable way of framing rights talk and of erecting plausible boundaries for individual sovereignty. In chapter 7 I will try to flesh out how respect for autonomy readily can accommodate relational concerns through the use of dialogue. Still, I will contend that patients' autonomous PSR decisions should be treated as inviolable.

Objections and Responses

There are a number of ways one might resist the above conclusion. First, one might object that autonomy and its exercise do not occupy the central place in our value system I have claimed. Second, one might argue that "minor incursions" on a patient's right to make PSR decisions need not, and moreover do not, destroy the conception of an autonomous being we wish to hold. Third, one might concede that personal sovereignty exists, but believe that the boundaries I have drawn are inappropriate. That is, one could hold that PSR decisions do exist and that individuals do have the right to make them, but argue that the range of such decisions is much narrower than I have suggested. This may be because few decisions actually qualify as PSR or, alternatively, because the designation PSR depends on the circumstances. For example, one might claim that suicide loses its PSR status, and hence sovereignty does not apply, if suicide would cause tremendous psychological injury to one's young children.[13] Note that this last line of argument is limited to "concern for others," as I have already argued that concern for future selves cannot override concern for one's present self.

In response to the first objection, that the value of autonomy and its exercise is not in fact as central as I suggest, I would point to the deep sense of betrayal and indignation that most people feel, even after years have passed, at their being prevented from making a decision that was PSR. This is not to say people do not come to terms with and perhaps even appreciate the results of having been denied.[14] But the sense of profound injustice remains. A particularly well-documented case involved Dax Cowart, who was forced to undergo extremely painful treatment for severe burns rather than be allowed to die.[15] Despite impressive recovery, a subsequent law degree, and a successful marriage, Cowart actively resents having been denied his sovereignty and maintains that he was done an extreme wrong. I contend that this reaction is both the norm and represents an important deep intuition that what we *do* and not merely what happens is morally important.[16] Unlike other common psychological reactions, moral indignation over being denied the right to make PSR decisions appeals to our conception of what it is to be a moral equal in society. In that sense I think it speaks quite strongly to the central value we place on autonomy and its exercise.

The second objection, that "minor incursions" on a patient's right to make PSR decisions are sufficiently benign to be overlooked, misunderstands the nature of what is at stake. Sovereignty and what it stands for is an all-or-nothing concept. Minor violations show the same disregard and disrespect for a person's status as a moral equal as do major violations. In terms of respecting my sovereignty, it makes no difference whether you tie me up for an hour just to see what I look like bound in twine or whether you hog-tie me with rope for a week. Nor does it matter that you restrain me to do me some good, for the crux of the issue is whether I have consented to your constraints. At times you may need to intervene to determine whether I am in fact autonomous, but that is a different matter.

A variation on this second objection combines the claim that minor incursions are insignificant with a "real self" argument, such as Danny Scoccia's that (paternalistic) intervention is justifiable when Sally's choice does not accurately express the desires she would have if she were fully rational.[17] Here the claim is "It's no big deal, and if Sally really thought about it, she'd agree with me." But tempting as this combined approach is, it both misunderstands the nature of respect for sovereignty and demands too much consistency to accommodate human behavior. If we respect a patient's choices *only* when they appear to be in her best interest, are prudent, or (even) consistent, it is not respect for sovereignty we exhibit. Moreover, if our standard for sovereignty demanded absolute consistency, such a move would license infinite interventions. For example, how could we reconcile a patient's underlying value for health with her decision to smoke cigarettes, eat red meat, or work fourteen-hour days? Respecting Sally's right to make PSR decisions means that *so long as we believe she is autonomous* no inconsistency, however flagrant, permits unwanted intervention, however minor. Various relationships may bend the boundaries of what constitutes intervention, but the principle remains unchanged. To demand less would fail to treat patients as self-governing moral equals.

The third objection, challenging whether many decisions in fact qualify as PSR or retain their PSR status inviolably, is harder to respond to. In preceding sections I have neither attempted to specifically catalogue which matters are PSR nor set out necessary and sufficient conditions for PSR status. Though I am not greatly concerned to carry out either of these practical tasks here, I do recognize that this incompleteness has the potential to severely undercut the force of my argument. That is, if it can be successfully argued that genuine instances of PSR decisions are rare, my practical aim will be defeated despite the success of the argument. At least at this point I am not prepared to list decisions that should be considered PSR, though it seems to me that the kinds of decisions I mentioned earlier—whether to commit suicide or refuse medical treatment or endanger oneself—are indeed paradigms of PSR decisions.

In terms of my position, perhaps the more problematic issue is whether circumstances exist in which something like the decision to commit suicide loses its PSR status. Consider two cases: First, imagine that a forty-year-old man decides, after considerable thought, deliberation, and consultation with others, that he no longer values life and wants to commit suicide. He is aware that his death will bring great suffering to the lives of his wife, children, parents, brothers, and sisters and that the interpersonal conflict and blaming that will go on after his death may cause significant family disruption. Second, imagine the same scenario but that the man's decision to kill himself is motivated by his desire to bring about the suffering and disruption of his family. Is it realistic to argue that either of these cases should count as PSR? Given my arguments so far, I am inclined to think that both cases would count as PSR and should be respected as such. But I am ill at ease with this conclusion, especially in the latter case.

Clearly, there are two sides to the matter. On the one hand, there are good reasons to take into account the consequences of otherwise quite private actions. As a community, we have a responsibility to protect the well-being of those around us when society is threatened. In fact it is just this sort of argument that Mill advanced regarding the degenerative effects of widespread (though essentially private) drunkenness, that when private actions so tear apart the fabric of society (or threaten to) they may rightfully be prohibited. On the other hand, in addition to significant shortcomings these "greater good" formulations have underlying problems. The shortcomings have to do with how "society" gets defined. Is a marriage a society? Is a family? What is the proper circumference of concern that allows for intervention, that transforms the personal into the political? Can we forcibly *include* within our sphere those (e.g., certain KKK factions) who deny membership to any larger society, and who thus demand to be free of our responsibility/right to intervene in their affairs? Perhaps more fundamentally, what constitutes "tearing apart" the fabric of society? I am reasonably convinced that such a charge would have been levied against the likes of Copernicus or Darwin or Ghandi or King. And this strikes me as deeply problematic. In particular, the suggestion that something can count as PSR *only* if no great suffering or strife would result is extremely problematic.

For the exercise of autonomy to survive as a meaningful concept there must be a way to define PSR matters such that the designation is not entirely dependent upon how others are affected.[18] For to do otherwise is to allow society to dictate the meaning that Sally's actions should have for her and thereby severely limit the sphere of actions Sally has the right to undertake without interference. If Irving's plan to marry outside the Jewish faith can be interfered with because of its destructive effect on the community, what meaningful sense of self-governance survives? I have argued that autonomy and its exercise stand as a fundamental, central value, and that by intervening in PSR matters we take away the dignity and respect that sustain our very conception of other human beings as moral equals. But for this conception of autonomy to be itself meaningful, *PSR* must be defined in a sufficiently broad manner to allow human beings some significant extent of control over their lives. Difficult cases like the ones described above seriously challenge our conception of PSR. But assuming these cases do qualify as PSR, I contend that our conception of what it is to be a moral equal demands that autonomous individuals be accorded the right to have the final say. Kant held that there are ways of treating a person that are inconsistent with recognizing her as a full member of the human community, and that such treatment is profoundly unjust.[19] We do not believe that it is right to treat a person unjustly simply to avoid suffering, even great public suffering. So why should public suffering dictate the boundaries for the legitimate exercise of self-government (assuming, of course, that the action wrongs no others)? This said, it may well be that there is no overarching principle for defining PSR matters, and the only solution is to deal with problematic situations on a case-by-case basis.

Further Reasons to Safeguard PSR Autonomous Decisions

There is, of course, also a variety of more pragmatic reasons for safeguarding a patient's right to make PSR decisions. First, assuming that in many cases there would need to be some institutional mechanism for overriding patients' decisions, institutions would be accorded the political and legal authority to carry out that overriding. But, given the political, racial, and other biases inherent in virtually any institution, we may well wish to avoid legally sanctioning unavoidably biased bureaucratic institutions to (paternalistically) override patients' PSR decisions.[20]

Second, and relatedly, people empowered by society to (paternalistically) override patients' PSR decisions will probably have more wealth, education, and political power than the average patient. For these reasons, it is likely that an intellectual, expert-oriented elitism will arise regarding what sorts of decisions actually get overridden and which populations get subjected to such overrides. I take it for granted that such intellectualist bias is undesirable.[21]

Third, because human beings do hold conflicting values, it is unreasonable and impractical to demand as a condition for not interfering with patients' PSR decisions that patients' choices always be consistent with their underlying values, and in particular their underlying value for health. But of course it is precisely such inconsistency that is used to justify much intervention. The difficulty with such justifications is that they seem unable to distinguish legitimate intervention from that which is illegitimate. Conflict, alone, cannot be sufficient to sanction overriding a patient's PSR decisions. For we can expect that autonomous choices often will conflict with *some* underlying value.

Fourth, it seems to me that respecting an individual's right to make PSR decisions forces individuals to take more responsibility for their own lives. In making this point I do not mean to suggest that individuals must shoulder all responsibility, for clearly individuals often find themselves in circumstances largely beyond their control. In fact it would be irresponsible to dismiss structural and sociological critiques that show how institutions and social structures create the oppressive and unjust conditions that contribute to and often precipitate the actions we ascribe to individuals. Nonetheless I would argue that insofar as we allow individuals to make their own PSR decisions, however foolish, unencumbered[22] by the "better judgment" of society, we thereby encourage them to take more control of their lives. Many problems in society would abate should we find a way to get individuals to take more responsibility, and thereby more control. In this sense, respecting patients' autonomous PSR decisions may play an important part in a much larger social and political picture.

An interesting question and possible challenge to my position about respecting PSR autonomous decisions is raised in connection with child geniuses. In most respects many child geniuses would qualify as autonomous on my scheme, and yet experience tells us that these individuals are nonetheless children, immature, and needing guidance and restrictions to help make them responsible decision-makers. Does this mean that there ought to be some dispositional or maturity component to autonomy? Self-interest, alone, makes me leery of such a criterion. More generally, though, I am not convinced that any acceptable set of dispositional qualities could be defined. That is, given the diversity found in society it is not at all clear what characterization of "maturity" could reasonably serve as a necessary condition for qualifying as autonomous.[23]

Perhaps a more enlightened response is to be found in Gerald Dworkin's view that "autonomy is a term of art introduced by a theorist in an attempt to make sense of a tangled net of intuitions, conceptual and empirical issues, and normative claims." Because Dworkin does not believe that we can "specify necessary and sufficient conditions without draining [autonomy] of the very complexity that enables it to perform its theoretical role," he argues that we should seek to characterize rather than define autonomy.[24] Thus one might argue that any characterization of autonomy must be flexible enough to acknowledge that various conditions for qualifying as autonomous must remain essentially undefinable. Hence there might be various undefinable developmental characteristics whose absence in even the brightest of children defines autonomy as a characteristic of adults. The essentially ad hoc nature of this response, however, makes me think either that we simply have yet to identify what is lacking in these children such that they should not be thought autonomous or that the appropriate response is to regard child geniuses as autonomous and treat them accordingly. In any event, I leave this as something to think about.

Conclusion

I have argued that we should think of autonomy as a threshold capacity and that because of its central place within our value system we should respect as sovereign patients' autonomous PSR decisions. Clearly a variety of often complex factors are involved in determining whether a person qualifies as autonomous. And because of this there will be times when (what turn out to be) autonomous desires must be overridden long enough to establish a person's autonomous status. Looking at decisions, per se, I have suggested that at base the process of decision-making is a black box and that the most we can do toward establishing the autonomy of a decision is to look at the conditions under which the decision was made. Proper analysis will encompass both psychological and environmental factors. But I have argued there is no reason to think that a person's autonomy cannot be expressed in choices that are decidedly foolish and even inconsistent with various underlying values. Such autonomous choices may constitute radical departures from a patient's characteristic behavior, and, as was the case with Alan, they may risk irreversible injury and even death. Nevertheless, I have claimed that, barring some autonomy-defeating condition, such choices are a patient's own to make.

It is, of course, our prerogative to say that some PSR autonomous decisions are tragic. But I think it is short-sighted and ultimately inconsistent with our deeply held values regarding autonomy to not respect PSR autonomous decisions. Given the nature of what it means to act out of respect for a person's autonomy, I have argued that it is at the very least misguided to claim that temporary indignities are defensible so long as they sufficiently promote the interests of those interfered with. Calls such as Mark Siegler's to shift the question from Where should decision-making power reside? to What is the right and good decision for this particular person in these particular circumstances? miss the point entirely.[25] For while it is good to promote a broader conversation, to widen (for Siegler) clinical decision-making strategies so they can account for greater spheres of knowledge and allow for a more holistic understanding of what is at issue in a particular decision, it simply is wrong to suggest that a decision that overrides a patient's PSR autonomous decision can yet be "the right and good decision."

Unfortunately, even quite reasoned discussions commonly fail to realize what is at stake in situations involving PSR decisions of autonomous individuals. Often, the reason is that attempts to get "beyond paternalism and autonomy" tend to ignore the fact that someone has to, i.e., gets to, make the final decision.[26] They ignore that sovereignty admits of no middle ground and that one must either pledge allegiance to respecting a person's autonomy or commit oneself to something else, be it medical efficiency, health, stability, happiness, or something else. It is not only that a person's status as a moral equal stands in the balance; there are also important social and political implications. Policy standards for whole classes of people in our society are at stake. Moreover, so long as we demean patients' abilities to decide how they will live their own lives, we cannot be surprised when they fail to take on individual responsibility or seem disinterested in developing their own capacities. It is unrealistic to expect people to aspire to autonomous lives when at the same time we judge them incapable of directing their lives. Though trite, it is clear: you get what you pay for.

Obviously, it is not always easy to recognize affronts to individuals' PSR autonomous decisions, as many disputes are wrapped up in other concerns, such as public safety, professional obligation, fiscal policy, and so on. When we do recognize such affronts, tragic outcomes can perhaps be avoided through education and dialogue. Presumably, we even have moral duties to engage in such activity that arise out of our professional responsibilities as well as our relationships with other human beings. But I hope I have been able to argue convincingly that when push comes to shove, it is our moral responsibility to respect the PSR autonomous wishes of individuals. For those, like Dr. J, who think the cost of respecting autonomy is too dear, I hope my arguments at least give pause, if not rebuttal.

⑦ The Landscape of Autonomy

Both as a community and as individuals, we often seek to help others live better, happier, more fulfilling lives. Not only do we give of ourselves and our resources but we also create policies and institutions and undertake actions and projects of all sorts intended to benefit others. There are, however, important ethical constraints on how we may attempt such altruism. Respect for the principle of justice, for example, prohibits us from exploiting the poor or forcing experimentation on the elderly or denying civil rights to criminals, even when such actions would benefit untold numbers of people. In part, the idea is that we have no right to use another person merely as a means to an end, however laudable that end happens to be. It is my position that a similar constraint is found in respect for the principle of autonomy. Specifically, I have contended that it is wrong to override a person's autonomous PSR decisions for paternalistic reasons. In this chapter I will attempt to reconcile this rather principlist claim with the relational concerns that attend clinical medicine. I will explain how one can both appreciate the full dynamics of a clinical situation and yet hold that patients' autonomous preferences should serve as a trump card in PSR matters, even when we think those preferences constitute bad choices for the agent. Additionally, I will try to show that respecting an autonomous decision involves entering into a relationship, a process that itself can be seen as educational.

Of course, HCPs have long wrestled with the tension between their professional assessments of clinical situations and patients' decisions about their own care. Medical decisions are virtually the paradigm for PSR decisions, and yet social and professional norms (on a variety of different levels) have resisted fully engaging patients with regard to the care they will receive. Some of this recalcitrance may be explained by paternalistic attitudes, and some no doubt by the entrenched biases or logistical barriers that attend medicine. But no small part is also due to a frequently superficial appreciation of patients' views combined with a fundamental misunderstanding about what it means to respect patients' autonomy.

Summary of Autonomy

I have characterized personal autonomy as a threshold concept comprising three general attributes: continuity of the self, a minimum (normative) standard of value, and procedural rationality. I take it as given that to be considered self-governing, Sally must exhibit some substantial psychological overlap in terms of memory, beliefs, habits, feelings, and so forth. Additionally, I have argued that Sally must embrace some intersubjectively accepted set of goods—e.g., certain powers and opportunities, rights and liberties, material resources, knowledge, self-respect. For were Sally to reject *all* such goods and instead consistently value pain, disability, poverty, misery, ignorance, limited freedom, and humiliation, it would be virtually impossible to make sense of her goals. In fact, unless Sally embraces some intersubjectively accepted set of goods, her notion of critical evaluation itself will be virtually incomprehensible to us. Lastly, I have argued that to be considered autonomous Sally must possess procedural rationality, for which she must embrace basic logical rules of inference and have the ability to formulate, revise, and pursue ends or goals in an intelligible manner. Integral to this ability is the capacity to deliberate, that is, to examine one's beliefs, desires, habits, values, and be able to recognize both evidence and inferences as compelling reasons for changing one's beliefs and behaviors. To be considered autonomous Sally must be able to raise the question of whether she will identify with or reject the reasons for which she now acts. She must understand that her decisions are open to critical reflection and, in turn, be capable of performing that examination in a procedurally independent manner.

I also have suggested that autonomy generally be regarded as a diachronic property, that is, as something possessed over time rather than located in particular decisions. A practical reason for holding this view has to do with the difficulty in making the sorts of qualitative distinctions necessary for determining which factors are most influential in generating a particular decision. Imagine, for example, how difficult it would be to figure out how much Sally's decision, say, to purchase a Maserati sports car is influenced by her actual assessment of the car, as opposed to the language used by the salesman, the showroom environment, Sally's preconceptions about being a Maserati owner, or even Sally's mood at the time of her decision. In addition to this basic inaccessibility, focusing on individual decisions risks overly narrow assessments of what should count as autonomous. For decisions that appear nonrepresentative at first blush may assume a very different character when viewed in a larger context. Now and again we may be concerned to determine whether some particular decision was autonomous or not, particularly when that decision would cause Sally great and irrevocable harm. But as with a painting the general focus should not be on each individual brushstroke. In fact I have tried to establish that to treat Sally as an autonomous being demands a certain flexibility, a willingness to accommodate her own interpretation and response to a given situation so long as she possesses the capacity for autonomy.

Concerning the value of autonomy, I have argued that it is the presumption of the capacity for autonomy that makes possible our conception of a full-fledged member of human society, that it is because Sally is presumed autonomous that her actions have the meaning for us that they do. The sorts of relationships we establish with Sally, how we interact with her, what we expect from her, what we conceive of as her responsibilities and her due, and even ontologically what constitutes her domain, all depend upon whether we conceive of Sally as an autonomous being. I have argued that autonomy is in fact a necessary condition for conceiving of others as our moral equals, of taking seriously their ideas and values and aspirations. And I have suggested that to give up this conception of individuals as autonomous beings is to lose hold of our orientation toward the world. For without the assumption that people have the capacity to formulate their own ideas, to assess and revise and endorse higher order plans and beliefs and values, how can we tie moral value or significance to people's actions? How can we ground the personal and institutional expectations that form the basis for the functioning of society? Education would become conditioning; justice, merely some homeostatic mechanism; achievement, an empty designation.

I have argued that because autonomy functions as a precondition for our conception of a full-fledged member of human society, to treat Sally as if she were *not* autonomous is to deny her status as a moral equal. Moreover, so long as we believe Sally is autonomous, treating her as an autonomous being and as a moral equal entails respecting her PSR decisions even when we believe those decisions are not in her best interest. For to respect Sally's choices only when we think them prudent is not to treat her as the author of her own life, but as a means that can be devalued when it no longer conduces to the end we desire. Because of this relationship I will speak interchangeably of respect for autonomy and respect for its exercise as I now turn to discuss a model for respecting autonomy.

Respecting Autonomy

Consider the following scenario. Leo, who is seventy-one years old, is told by his nurse practitioner, Shaun, that he probably has prostate cancer. Shaun explains that Leo's prostate specific antigen is acutely elevated and that a biopsy would cement the diagnosis and allow them to initiate appropriate treatment. Over the course of about twenty minutes of questioning by Leo, Shaun explains that treatment likely would begin with hormone therapy followed by either surgery or radiation therapy. Because Leo is concerned about possible side effects, Shaun explains that Leo is liable to develop some secondary female sex characteristics from the hormone therapy (e.g., enlarged breasts, loss of body hair) and that surgery might induce urinary incontinence and even sexual impotence. Shaun explains that if the cancer is caught early enough cure is virtually assured, but that without treatment Leo should not expect to live more than about ten years.

Leo, who is widowed and lives with his daughter and her family, calmly but somewhat aggressively refuses any further diagnostic or therapeutic treatment. He requests that Shaun just drop the matter entirely and further directs Shaun not to tell anyone else about his condition. Leo wishes Shaun to continue to monitor his blood pressure (for which he takes medication) and to continue providing him medical care as needed, but to stay out of his business as far as his prostate is concerned. Upon being pressed, Leo explains that he just wants to live out his life as God intended him to and to die "naturally" and with the dignity he has always had. Leo then tells Shaun that he is tired, does not want to talk about it anymore, and will see Shaun the following month, thank you very much.

Assuming that Leo is autonomous and that Shaun is conscientious, there clearly is a dilemma here. Without some (apparently unwanted) intervention, Leo seems fated to suffer a preventable premature death that likely will be painful and prolonged.[1] And yet, Shaun has been presented with a clear, firm request. Shaun has been told by an autonomous patient not to intervene in his affairs, at least with regard to his prostate condition. Having overseen Leo's medical care for the past two years, Shaun feels a sense of responsibility for Leo's well-being not just as an HCP but also as someone who truly cares for him. Because prostate cancer is notoriously slow growing, Shaun does have some time to maneuver. Delaying treatment by a month or two probably will not change the prognosis significantly. But what should Shaun do?

Given the prevailing norms within the Western practice of medicine and that this is a PSR matter, the answer seems clear: Shaun should respect Leo's decision. End of story? Well, not exactly. The reason is that it is not entirely clear what it *means* to respect Leo's autonomous decision, what it involves and what it precludes. Though often overlooked by advocates of the primacy of respect for autonomy as well as detractors, respecting autonomous decisions neither implies accepting pronouncements at face value nor precludes asking questions.[2] A statement's face value may not effectively communicate the intended or underlying meaning, if only because the HCP misunderstands it. By asking questions we often can better understand the nature of a decision and the reasoning behind it. And presumably the more we know, the better equipped we will be to respect that decision.

There are, of course, any number of reasons to *not* ask questions. A statement's meaning may seem entirely clear or the decision may seem sufficiently inconsequential as to not be worth investigating further. Alternatively, due to either ignorance or negligence, one might be simply unaware that ambiguity is possible. Other times callous disregard or even ignominious intent may explain the failure to investigate. So, for example, one might accept Leo's decision to ignore his prostate condition because one did not care about Leo or perhaps had something to gain by accepting the face value of his pronouncement. Still further, structural barriers can intervene, such as time constraints or language barriers or even statutory prohibitions against asking questions.

The point, however, is that though sometimes there is no alternative but to accept statements at face value and though sometimes this does not result in misunderstanding, without real communication one cannot presume to know how to respect another person's autonomous decisions. Embedded in this observation is the kernel of what it means to respect a patient's autonomous decision. For what is implied by this recognition that *understanding is the cornerstone of respecting autonomous decisions* is that respecting someone's autonomous decision involves entering into a relationship with that person, however brief. In other words, respecting Leo's autonomous decision involves having a genuine appreciation of what Leo actually wants. But this requires *either* that shared networks of understanding already exist that are "sufficiently full" *or* that we engage in some sort of communicative process that brings about such mutual understanding. Lacking a shared understanding, the most we can do is respect what we presume to be Leo's autonomous decision, a presumption that may be as mistaken as a first guess at charades.

It is important to recognize that engaging in such a communicative process is not just relational but educational in that it encourages us to more fully examine our own selves and our understanding of the world. For in seeking to understand another we come to terms with her beliefs, practices, and values by drawing connections between them and our own. To the extent that communicative interactions are geared toward mutual understanding, then, they provide us the educational opportunity to develop a deeper appreciation of who we are and what we believe. Of course, not all decisions are of the same moment nor is their educational potential identical. Depending on their importance, a patient's decisions will command different levels of concern on our part. The more at stake the greater reason we have to want to understand the nature of the decision we mean to honor as autonomous. Hence, Leo's decision to ignore a potentially fatal (and curable) condition likely will engage us more deeply than would Leo's decision to, say, ignore his seasonal allergies.

It is worth noting that in the real world of clinical medicine patient decisions are more likely to be questioned—either for clarification or to challenge their autonomous nature—when they run contrary to an HCP's personal judgment. On one level this is certainly troubling insofar as it implies that inquiries regarding autonomy can be used as pretenses for effecting power plays, for controlling and circumventing patients' wishes. On another level, however, it is quite understandable that HCPs should challenge those decisions that do not seem right to them. As people whose business it is to provide care in order to promote the health of others, it is nothing less than responsible for HCPs to seek to understand more fully decisions that conflict with their own estimation of what is in the patient's best interest. What is unclear, of course, is the extent to which HCPs have a responsibility to investigate patients' pronouncements, to engage in a dialogue to clarify meaning. How far must they push to ensure a genuine understanding of the patient's wishes? Though in part this is an empirical matter, it is also a normative question whose answer depends on how one views the relationship between a patient and an HCP.

That HCPs' roles are defined (largely) in terms of promoting health and preventing harm provides a basis for gauging HCPs' responsibilities to engage in the kind of dialogical relationship sometimes necessary for realizing mutual understanding. For the greater the potential of a given health care decision to affect a patient's health, the more it invokes the health-promoting role of HCPs, and hence the greater the imperative to ensure that a shared genuine understanding has been reached.[3] The way to reach this understanding, I will suggest, is *dialogue,* whose value and promise lie in its potential to help individuals transcend otherness. For dialogue is a form of relationship that engages individuals in a deep and reciprocal interaction whose goal is to examine and establish interconnections. In this sense dialogue is inherently developmental, enabling its participants to more fully understand how their perceptions, beliefs, values, and practices relate to each other and to the world at large. This sort of integration thus establishes dialogue as an educational encounter and in many ways grounds its value as a relation that can help HCPs understand what respecting a patient's autonomous decision means in any given situation. For at base dialogue aims to overcome barriers that separate people, preventing their mutuality.

It is of little consequence that such unity is elusive, if not by definition unrealizable. For dialogue must be understood as a developmental process that is both enriching in its own right and strategically valuable. In terms of respecting autonomous decisions, dialogue establishes for HCPs an avenue for helping resolve misunderstandings, mediate conflicts, promote patients' interests (including patients' exercise of autonomy and sense of empowerment), and even question a patient's capacity for autonomy. Clearly, the nature of particular patient-HCP relationships will help define what is possible and what is expected from particular interactions. Relationships that are superficial and perfunctory and disjunct generally will have very different parameters for interaction than those that are long-standing, broad-based, well-developed, and intimate. Because relationships are not static but instead form and adapt (intentionally as well as due to circumstance and necessity), any given patient-HCP relationship will exhibit different levels of intimacy, commitment, and so forth at different points in time. Presumably, the deeper and more well-established the relationship the greater basis exists for pushing hard, for assuming a greater responsibility to engage in dialogue, and for achieving a shared understanding. Still, clear boundaries will seldom emerge. Often HCPs will have no choice but to guesstimate the latitude that various relationships demand and allow in terms of working to develop a deep understanding of their patient's decision.

It is in part precisely this indeterminateness that makes contractual models of health care so attractive to some HCPs. It is assumed that by framing the professional interaction as a fixed bill of exchange rather than as a relationship whose terms and interaction must be negotiated the guesswork is removed regarding one's professional responsibilities for coming to understand and deal with the patient. Clearly, contracts do help set more definitive boundaries regarding professional responsibilities. However, unless *all* aspects of professional relationships are to be standardized and *all* patient statements are to be taken at face value, some communicative interaction still will play an integral part in determining the boundaries of any given situation. And it is this realization that points to the importance of dialogue. Imagine, for example, that Sally goes to Planned Parenthood and requests the most effective means of birth control. It is simply not reasonable to accept this statement at face value without engaging Sally further. Presumably, a hysterectomy is the most effective means of birth control. But before it even makes sense to provide the best reversible treatment, all sorts of questions need to be asked about Sally's past medical history, possible allergies, underlying beliefs, and so forth. Relying on face value to interpret patient decisions does not reflect the diagnostic nature of promoting health and also ignores that unless one is careful to investigate sources of possible misunderstanding misconceptions can abound even in the most familiar and seemingly straightforward situations. And this describes just the surface level. Clearly, the goal is not to question every assumption, but to ignore the existence of otherness entirely is to be either amazingly unaware or particularly uncaring. To genuinely respect patients' autonomous decisions, it is imperative that HCPs enter into relationships with patients and moreover recognize that oftentimes they will need to engage in dialogue to create a sense of shared understanding.

Putting Respect for Autonomy in Context

We can now describe how Shaun might go about respecting Leo's autonomous (PSR) decision regarding his prostate condition in a way that also promotes Leo's well-being. Assuming that a viable patient-HCP relationship exists, Shaun has a responsibility to try to engage Leo in a dialogue. Working within the parameters of the relationship they have developed, Shaun then can inquire into Leo's reasoning. Is he scared of sexual and urinary dysfunction? Is he ashamed of his condition? What does Leo mean by dying "naturally" and with dignity? Is Leo confused about what prostate cancer means for him medically or financially or socially? Does Leo need/want reassurance? guidance? more information? or simply time to process the news? Shaun might even inquire about the parameters of their dialogue. For example, should Leo refuse to discuss his condition altogether, Shaun might ask why he is so reticent or whether Leo would be willing to discuss the matter with someone else.

For better or worse, Shaun has few clear guidelines for how to proceed in this dialogue. There will be no objective way to determine which of Leo's responses should be accepted at face value and which should be questioned further. Because certain values and rationales are seen as constitutive of being rational, there are some general normative standards for gauging responses. In other words, responses that reflect values such as liberty, the absence of pain, feelings of self-respect, and so forth will be understandable prima facie and as such will help define the parameters of Shaun's inquiry. So, for example, were Leo to explain that he finds his existence a misery and does not want to prolong it, especially when doing so might significantly impair (what he considers) his masculinity, this would count as an "understandable" response that required no further inquiry. Clearly, there must be considerable flexibility for what counts as an understandable response, and in general Shaun will need to be sensitive to the context of the interaction. For dialogues are particular and their individual courses will depend upon their specific dynamics, including the nature of the relationship between the participants as well as the circumstances of the encounter.

That one must first understand a patient's decision to know how best to respect it explains why respecting autonomous decisions often involves engaging in dialogue.[4] Nothing in the characterization I have presented, however, suggests that respect for autonomy should be the sole reason for engaging in dialogue[5] or that other principles or motivations are not ingredient to encounters between patients and HCPs. In no way am I meaning to present respect for autonomy as a totalizing theory. Caring and beneficence will find their way into virtually all HCPs' interactions with patients; and so, too, other principles such as justice, nonmaleficence, utility, mercy, and so forth will have their application. Still, I have argued that the principle of respect for autonomy defines the outer boundaries for what HCPs may do.

By regarding patients' autonomous decisions as the ultimate directive for scripting health care encounters between HCPs and patients (in PSR matters), and yet recognizing that self-governance must take place within a context defined by not only the circumstances of the interaction but also the dynamics of various relationships, the model I have presented bridges various surface differences between traditional and alternative approaches to ethical analysis. It is principlist insofar as it holds up respect for the exercise of autonomy (in PSR matters) as a nuclear principle that cannot be dismissed or abrogated for circumstantial reasons. That is, it holds firm that when dealing with autonomous patients the final structure for decision-making is independent of the particulars of the situation. But the model I have presented also takes up various feminist/relationist concerns challenging the rigidity of principlist approaches to ethics. Specifically, it recognizes that milieu, environment, and even the personalities of those involved in a given situation play a pivotal role in framing and dealing with an ethical conflict. In this model no issue or consideration is excluded from the ethical dialogue a priori or prevented from exerting its (rightful) influence with regard to the situation at hand.[6]

In a number of ways, the position I present reflects a kind of specified principlism.[7] But here "specification" refers to and involves the *process* of respecting autonomy, as opposed to a cumulative cataloging of specifications for how autonomy ought to be respected. In other words, my position holds that given the overarching principle of respect for autonomy (in PSR matters), specification of what it means to respect a person's autonomy should occur during each particular encounter in which respecting autonomy arises as an issue. And rather than being conceived of as a cumulative qualification of a fixed code, specification would concern and attempt to establish the direction and character that particular dialogues should take. By thus being conceived of as a process that is adaptable and sensitive to the particulars of situations and relationships, the principle of respect for autonomy (in PSR matters) can avoid rigid abstraction and yet retain its overriding importance. Moreover, by embracing dialogue the process of respecting autonomy engages HCPs in a critical, educational project. For dialogue calls on its participants to (re)examine assumptions and (re)draw the interconnections that comprise their understanding of otherness, their constructions of meaning.

A particular advantage of this dialogical model over other principlist approaches is that the discursive method for specifying what respecting autonomy means centers on negotiation, and as such is (or at least can be) less reliant on established traditions of right and wrong, good and bad. When the principle of respect for autonomy is applied and how it is adapted is not determined by coherence with some overall set of background norms in society, norms that we know to be steeped in a variety of biases. The dialogical method proposed here instead relies on only a minimal set of normative values—namely, those necessary to determine whether a person is autonomous and serve as guideposts for which sorts of statements and responses should be accepted at their face value. Moreover, the dialogical method proposed here allows the process of respecting the exercise of autonomy to be as inclusive as any given relationship can tolerate, or at least *wants* to tolerate. Virtually any concern can be raised in the course of dialogue so long as those engaged in the dialogue have a relationship that can accommodate those issues and considerations. As a result, this dialogical model can incorporate alternative viewpoints quite easily while staying within the principlist framework that holds firm to the primacy of respecting patients' exercise of autonomy (in PSR matters).

Because the position I present does not provide for some cumulative *summae* regarding what it means to respect autonomy, it is less directly tied to the casuistic method.[8] Like casuistry, my position does appreciate that our lives comprise a multidimensional matrix of beliefs and values and feelings. Like casuistry, it recognizes that the full store of life's experiences is relevant for framing and analyzing ethical conflict, and as such must be included in any dialogical process that aims to resolve conflict. But unlike casuistry, my position does not seek to establish a canon of maxims. Whereas casuistry would seek to establish a maxim for what it means to respect autonomy in situations (sufficiently) similar to situation A, and another maxim for B-like situations, the dialogical model I have presented does not go beyond the initial maxim that one should respect autonomy in PSR matters. In this model what it means (exactly) to respect autonomy will depend upon the nongeneralizable particulars of each and every situation, and as such must be left to negotiation. For it is understood that respecting autonomy is a process that develops out of the unique relations that exist between unique people. Clearly, the dialogical project of respecting autonomy in and through the development of greater *understanding* relies on the existence of commonly accepted interpretations and judgments. But at root such respect depends upon the irreducibly individual project of establishing interconnections, of *individuals* overcoming otherness by coming to terms with others rather than simply by acceding to the relevant maxim.

This focus on individuals is, however, both a strength and a weakness. As various feminist and relationist approaches to ethics are wont to point out, many of the problems we encounter in ethics, and certainly in bioethics, are rooted in institutional rather than individual practices. The difficulty with employing an institutional approach in the present context, however, is that it is not clear how respect for autonomy arises as a systemic concern, except insofar as particular institutional policies conflict with patients' autonomous PSR decisions. Suppose, for example, that the policy at Mount Sinai Hospital is that nurses must always defer to physicians' orders and that the hospital's staffing and priorities are such that there is seldom any opportunity for meaningful nurse-physician discussions about patient care. One can easily imagine that in such a context many of the conflicts involving respect for autonomy that arise between patients and nurses will be directly traceable to hospital policy. And yet it is problematic to address the hospital policy, itself, *in terms of* respect for autonomy. Now, this does not mean that Mount Sinai's policies are outside the scope of ethical inquiry and analysis, only that they cannot be addressed on the same terms as the immediate conflict. In other words, I agree with many feminists and relationists that it is arbitrary to select crisis issues as the only proper business of ethics when ethical conflicts can be identified just as easily with the more mundane "house-keeping issues" of habits and policies.[9] But I also believe that it is problematic to construe or resolve such house-keeping issues in terms of the arguments I have made regarding respect for autonomy in PSR matters.

Perhaps the way to address this institutional aspect is to deal with it as a developmental issue. That is, one might argue that as a society that values autonomy as centrally as we do we have certain responsibilities to promote and foster autonomy in those around us. Presumably, this would involve creating institutions and formulating policies that both facilitate autonomous decision-making and avoid (or prevent) conflicts that involve autonomy from arising in the first place. Such a concern for autonomy, combined with a general concern to avoid ethical conflict, might go a long way toward addressing the institutional and general house-keeping issues that are relevant to respecting autonomy.

In and of itself, the principle of respect for autonomy is not particularly sensitive to the sorts of process issues just mentioned. But unlike many traditional models for ethical inquiry and analysis, the dialogical model I have presented is inclusive by its very structure. Because the core notion of dialogue involves working to establish interconnections, it is not only able to accommodate any relevant issue but also intended to construct meaningful bridges between our understanding of conflict and the (full range of) conditions that give rise to it—some of which may include issues of gender, race, social class, power in general, even communication styles. What this points to is the critical and educational character of this model for respecting autonomy. For by being concerned with establishing meaningful relationships, the dialogical model I have presented aims to help HCPs develop a deeper and broader understanding of the nature and meaning of their beliefs, values, and practices—which, ideally, would also include a fuller understanding of the role of various institutional practices and values.

Additionally, it is important to recall that the dialogical model I have presented for respecting autonomy is inherently performance based. In this model, respecting Sally's autonomy depends upon having a deep understanding of her autonomous wishes, which in turn requires the ability to effect genuine communication. I think it is reasonable to assume that the sorts of communicative and investigational habits that make up such a (dialogical) process for respecting autonomy will lead to (if not themselves involve) the sorts of "house-keeping" practices that on both an individual and an institutional level help prevent ethical conflicts involving autonomy from arising in the first place. Indeed, it is a virtue of this model that it promotes the asking of questions, a habit that is aimed at understanding, at comprehending the situation so that one will be better able to further one's ultimate goals.

Obviously, this approach for respecting autonomy is rooted in the modern tradition and in that sense is quite rationalistic. Because such admissions nowadays seem to require some sort of qualification, I would just add that the dialogical principlist model I have presented is meant to be inclusive and constructive rather than restrictive. The premise that with greater levels of knowledge we will be better able to sort out our conflicts is not so naive, not so hopelessly romantic as many postmodernists paint it to be, if what we mean by knowledge is a full-bodied understanding and appreciation of people and their decisions, ideas, and plans. Unless one thinks that differences are inherently unresolvable, it is not naive to think that developing a genuine understanding of people moves us closer to understanding how to resolve the conflicts that arise out of our differences. It is in essence an educational belief, that by understanding our situation we can improve it, enrich it. And I, for one, am not convinced that any other view can hold out the promise of hope.

Concerns about the Principle of Respect for Autonomy

There are, of course, some other important concerns about this rather modernist approach. One particularly troubling matter is the relationist objection that it is artificial, if not dangerous, to draw the kinds of distinctions between people and their circles of interest that I have. In particular, it is argued that the designation PSR simply does not exist and that *all* decisions are fundamentally social. Strong relationists, as I will call them, claim that the very process of deliberation, judgment, choice, is so completely interpenetrated by our social interactions and context that the process of making decisions does not belong to anyone at all. One might conceive of it in the following way. The nature of a decision, combined with the particular circumstances in which it arises, describes what can be thought of as an area of immediate involvement surrounded by a series of increasingly distant concentric circles of association. Those individuals found within the inner radius have a greater role to play in dealing with the matter at hand than those found at the periphery *because* the former stand in closer relation to the matter at hand. On this strong relational model, waves of involvement ripple outward from a decision. So, while deciding what constitutes a near or distant relation may well involve some degree of interpretation, the claim of involvement is seen as an empirical matter.[10] From this it follows that whether a decision is properly someone's concern is not a function of some a priori designation, but is determined by looking at who is affected by a decision and how.

So, for example, consider the previous scenario with Leo, who has prostate cancer. Imagine now that Leo's son-in-law, Nate, overhears the very end of Leo and Shaun's original conversation. After speaking with Leo but getting no real information, Nate tells his wife, May, about his suspicion that something is wrong with Leo. Because Leo will not tell May anything either, May then seeks out Shaun to learn what is going on. May, who is a strong relationist, explains to Shaun that as Leo's daughter she is proximally situated to the center of most matters that concern Leo and as such deserves to be a part of any decision-making process about her father's health care. After all, May is Leo's only immediate relative, and more than that they live in the same house.[11]

In evaluating this strong relational claim, it is important not to confuse an ethical mandate with simply being considerate or kind. It is one thing to say that Leo should be more considerate of others by allowing those who care for him to play a role in this situation. It is quite another to say that, ethically speaking, it is not up to Leo whom to include in the decision-making process, but rather that the scope of involvement will itself depend upon the specific context of the decision. It is the latter claim that strong relationists wish to make and that those of us concerned to establish the primacy of respecting the exercise of autonomy in PSR matters must rebut.

Perhaps the place to begin a response is with the metaphor of concentric circles and what counts as a more proximate relation. On what basis is proximity to be judged? Presumably, there are no formal criteria such as being a family member or an old friend. One may be estranged from one's family; recent friendships may be deeper and more meaningful than longstanding ones; one may feel more interconnected with someone one knows professionally or formally (e.g., a therapist) than with one's social companions. In fact, the people we know enjoy variable proximities for different concerns and aspects of our lives, sometimes inhabiting an inner circle, sometimes a more distant one. In this respect, the strong relationist is right to claim that who counts as a proximate relation will depend upon context.

But of course one cannot define proximity simply in terms of ramifications. To use consequences as the measure for whether someone stands in close relation to a decision and hence deserves to have a prominent role in the decision-making process is extremely problematic. In purely practical terms it would prove both cumbersome and contentious to require a thorough accounting of all the major ramifications before one could identify who should be included in any given decision-making process. But more importantly, it is not clear that simply being affected by a decision should give a person power regarding how that decision is made. By way of illustration, consider the following two examples. Imagine that Camille is deciding whether to leave her current managerial position for a better one at another firm. If Camille leaves, Jake, a known misogynist, would take her place, to the great misfortune of Camille's fellow workers, especially Karen, who would have to work with Jake frequently and intimately. Though we may wish to say that Camille ought to take these consequences into consideration in making her decision, surely there is something wrong about the notion that Camille's decision actually *belongs* in part to Karen. Consider a second scenario in which a hospitalized patient, Daniel, provides the perfect opportunity for his longtime physician, Margaret, to test a particular treatment hypothesis of hers. The treatment has virtually no risk involved and if correct would catapult Margaret into international prominence in her field. We may wish to argue that as a longtime friend and patient Daniel should weigh the importance of this small commitment on his part against the meaning it would have for Margaret. We may wish to argue that it behooves Daniel to consider what his decision will mean for their relationship. But it is, again, quite another matter to claim that the decision *is* partly Margaret's. To define proximate relations by reference to consequences is to allow all decision-making processes to devolve into a political struggle. For to deserve a role in decision-making, all that a person would need to show is that she is affected by that decision. On this reading, the more a person is affected, the more the decision belongs to her. But this would mean that no decision, however personal, could be immune from the influence of those whose interests it would effect. I take the strength of this critique to be sufficiently obvious that it need not be pursued further to demonstrate the severe difficulties associated with using consequences to define proximate relations.[12]

Of course, a strong relationist might respond that, indeed, the matter of inclusion in the decision-making process is not about consequences, but rather is about relationships. Unlike the consequences model, on which all that matters is the extent to which one is affected by a decision, here it is argued that what is relevant is the extent to which a relationship exists and is meaningful. On this reading, the whole concept of ownership of a decision is rejected. Relationships just exist and to appreciate a relationship is to recognize that membership in the relationship entails some role in decision-making insofar as a particular decision concerns interests relevant to one's membership in the relation. In other words, relationships hold in specific contexts. And to the extent that a given relationship does hold and is meaningful, being in that relationship endows one with a role in making those decisions that affect the relationship.

In one sense, this is very egalitarian. It suggests that different forms of commitment (personal, intellectual, professional, and so forth) simply give rise to levels of participation commensurate with the depth of the relationship. Or to put it another way, the more meaningful and interconnected a relationship, the more of a role is created for each member in making decisions that concern that relationship. Thus, for example, Shaun would have more of a role in the decision concerning Leo's prostate condition than would a nurse practitioner who had not established a caring and meaningful relationship with Leo during the previous two years.

There are, however, a number of significant problems with using membership in a relationship to determine how decisions get made. First, how does it get decided which matters are of concern for a given relationship? Second, how is the depth of a relationship gauged? Relatedly, how broadly will involvement in decision-making range? To use the metaphor of concentric circles, how far out into the various ripples of association must participation extend?[13] Fourth, and perhaps most central for the process of decision-making, how can we differentiate relationships one from another? That is, is it possible to distinguish relationships into *kinds* so that only certain kinds of relationship depth, intimacy, and meaningfulness confer to someone a role in the decision-making process? If yes, then on what basis can such distinctions be made? If no, does this mean that so long as the depth and meaningfulness of the relationships are the same, one cannot distinguish between, say, the role one's spouse should play in making a decision versus the role one's therapist should play? If indeed such distinctions are not feasible, many if not all the distinctions we employ in society (public/private, professional/personal, formal/informal) would become unusable, a conclusion that is at the very least troubling.

Making Distinctions among Relationships

But assuming that some kinds of distinctions are possible, how do we make them? The nature of the strong relational model does not easily admit of any formal criteria for making distinctions between kinds of relationships— and this includes the possibility that criteria can be laid out in advance. Any mechanism for making distinctions will have to take into account competing views about what counts as a relationship "sufficiently close" to warrant significant involvement in a decision-making process. Any mechanism for drawing distinctions will have to deal with various power plays that attempt to establish certain forms of decision-making over others. The difficulty for the strong relational model, however, is that it is supposed to be nonhierarchical, which makes it problematic to appoint someone (or some body) judge or even arbiter over such matters. In other words, the strong relational model has a hard time dealing with competing interpretations of who should or should not participate in a decision-making process precisely because the strong relational model denies the existence of privileged interpretations. Of course, ideally these are the kinds of terms and arrangements that can be negotiated. But an equal part of the strong relationist claim is that, negotiation or not, relationships simply *do* convey/ entail a role in decision-making. And it is this assertion in the absence of any discursive mechanism that makes strong relationism both unrealistic and unacceptable as the basis for an actual model for decision-making.

For example, imagine that Leo refuses to tell May, Nate, the children, or anyone else about his condition despite their protestations that as people in close relationships with him any decision about his medical condition and care belongs to them, too. Unlike the dialogical process discussed earlier, with the strong relational position it is not at all clear on what terms negotiation or arbitration would proceed to shared decision-making. That is to say, here it is not apparent how to get beyond the initial impasse in a way that does not already privilege certain individuals by according them status as a (sufficiently) closely related member of a relationship. For if we are willing to override Leo's decision under the circumstances that have been described, then on what basis can *anyone* (assuming they claim to be closely related to the person and situation) be excluded from the decision-making process? If the strong relationist argument is right, then presumably there is no situation that Leo could keep to himself, nor is there a clear (or objective) way to differentially weigh individuals' relationship claims. Anyone in a relationship with Leo can claim to deserve a role in situations or decision-making processes that concern their relationship with Leo, and neither Leo nor anyone else will have any special power to exclude that person.

Unless someone (or some group) is given special power to decide which relationships belong in the inner radius and which should be located more distantly, and when, defining the boundaries/parameters for any particular decision will be intractably problematic. But what are the options for such authority? Certainly, majority vote will not do, for this would transform the ethics of decision-making into little more than a crass political activity. Appointing a judge to decide which relationships belong in which particular concentric circles is likewise problematic, since to do so would unfairly privilege someone's interpretation of relationships, and the point of the strong relationist view is that relationships entail certain involvements irrespective of how they are interpreted by others. Now, of course, there are formal legal mechanisms for such determinations. But, again, these will not do. For what is sought is a nonarbitrary mechanism for identifying which relationships, and more particularly which individuals, are important enough to be included in the process of decision-making.

In effect, strong relationists are aiming for a mechanism that is at once meaningful and able to distinguish amongst relationships, according to their significance. But it would seem that neither criteria nor individuals exist that can effect such a mechanism without unduly privileging some particular perspective over others. The way out of this dilemma lies in recognizing that, at bottom, meaning is subjective, arising out of the particular interconnections drawn between the phenomenon at issue and other reference points in the world. In virtually all cases this construction of meaning will be strongly influenced by culture and prevailing ideologies and may even be a thoroughly cooperative venture. Still, *someone* must draw the interconnections that give rise to meaning, and because of this the reference for meaning always must be *in terms of someone.* Thus, to meaningfully distinguish between relationships that confer a role in decision-making and relationships that do not, we must decide *in terms of whom* meaning should be construed, for whom such distinctions should be meaningful. The reason that this move is an escape from the strong relationist dilemma is that by acknowledging that *meaning* belongs to an interpretation rather than a situation, we are forced to identify whose interpretation, whose drawing of interconnections, should predominate. In that sense we are forced to choose between competing authors. We must decide whose voice should be granted the right to define what meaning different relationships have with regard to a particular situation.

Of course in many situations, if not most, no one voice may merit such overarching privilege. Shared responsibilities and privileges may locate the right to define meaning, the right to determine the regard that particular relationships deserve, in a broader population. Thus, despite having escaped from the strong relationist dilemma of *whether* particular interpretations should be privileged, in many cases we may still find ourselves at pains to reckon *whose* interpretations of meaning ought to be privileged. One of the great advantages of using a dialogical model for addressing the divisions between people is that dialogue provides a ready avenue for negotiating their different interpretations of the world. Because dialogue is in many senses directed toward mutual understanding, it is a process well suited for reaching shared interpretations of meaning. But part of what I have argued is that certain kinds of situations and decisions so fundamentally and thoroughly devolve on the individual that they deserve the designation PSR and in that sense should be defined in terms of the individual. It is, of course, difficult to establish in any absolute fashion that particular matters should be considered PSR. But to the extent that it is appropriate for the meaning of situations to be defined by and in terms of discrete groups of individuals, I have suggested that certain situations can be identified with single individuals and that it is in part the existence of such an inner sphere of issues that gives meaning to the notion of being the author of one's own life. Beyond encouraging the individual to draw her own interconnections, the importance of such dominion in terms of self-governance is that it allows the individual to evaluate the meaning and importance that her relations with the world will have for her.

Take Leo's situation as an example. The primary issue is the meaning that Leo's interconnections with the world should have, the value of a particular kind of existence for Leo, how Leo's life should go. Though May's and Shaun's concerns are relevant, it is not their lives, not their constructions of meaning that are at stake. But if this is so, who other than Leo should determine how much force the relationships and interconnections in his life should exert? Who is better situated than Leo to create meaning in (and out of) his life? At the end of the day someone has to make the final decision. Someone gets to draw the boundaries that distinguish the inner radius of human relationships from the outlying concentric circles of more distant association. What I am claiming is that in PSR matters so long as Leo possesses the capacity for autonomy there is no one other than Leo to whom we should grant that authority. For doing so not only would misplace the locus of meaning but also would, deny Leo the right to authorship that is constituent to being treated as a moral equal in society. This is not to say that others cannot or should not try to influence Leo's decisions. Shaun, for example, has every reason to engage Leo in dialogue, being both an HCP whose role is invoked by the seriousness of Leo's situation and someone who is in a meaningful relationship with Leo. As so often in health care, the vitality and complexity of Leo's situation places Shaun in a special and intimate position not only to better understand Leo and his decisions but also to help Leo develop a fuller understanding of his own beliefs, practices, and values by helping Leo explore alternative perspectives and interpretations, alternative ways to draw interconnections and construct meaning.

Clearly, the extent to which Shaun may push Leo in and through dialogue will depend on the nature and boundaries of their relationship, not to mention Shaun's own talent for dialogue. But in terms of respecting patients' autonomy, one sees in dialogue a particularly powerful model that is able to deal with many of the issues that make respecting autonomy complex and sometimes problematic. First and foremost, dialogue represents a process for dealing with otherness. By building on relationships dialogue can help HCPs develop a deeper understanding of what is involved in and entailed by a particular autonomous decision. Moreover, dialogue can function as an educational process that helps and pushes patients to clarify and develop the nature and meaning of their decisions. Dialogue is also a critical process in that virtually any belief, value, issue, or even dynamic can be called into question and examined, including whether a patient in fact possesses the capacity for autonomy. And yet also built into the dialogical model I have described is the notion that the purpose of engaging in dialogue is to better respect patients' autonomous decisions. For at the end of the day it is respect for patients' autonomy (in PSR matters) that must be given priority by HCPs.

Qualifications

As with so many things, of course, the tone expressed in championing autonomy often will be as important as the actual content of our position. In particular, we must make clear that despite various baggage[14] *respecting autonomy* constitutes an endorsement of neither rugged individualism nor self-absorption. It in no way entails an insensitivity or a lack of concern for personal relationships or for other factors integral to our lives. To view the position I have outlined as legitimizing exclusion is to mistake the principle for its abuse. There is no doubt that certain patients will use their right to exercise their autonomy in PSR matters to exclude others and will do so for selfish and perhaps even malicious reasons. But that certain individuals make poor use of their opportunities to forge interconnections with the world does not undermine the importance of respecting and safeguarding such opportunities. The point of the principle of respect for autonomy is that people should be allowed and encouraged to lead and develop their own lives as they see fit, to assume responsibility not just for directing their lives but also for creating meaning in (and out of) their lives. Given this understanding, respecting patients' exercise of autonomy in PSR matters is more than a progressive step forward, it is a prerequisite for encouraging individuals to take responsibility and develop themselves.

Another concern with the strong position I have taken is that in the current medical environment the imperative to respect patients' autonomous PSR decisions will be interpreted simply as an injunction to acquiesce to patients' expressed statements. For not only is there a natural tendency to oversimplify complex processes but also there is often neither time for the sorts of encounters I have described nor the underlying relationships necessary for carrying them out. Clearly, this is a danger. And yet studies have shown that it is both medically beneficial and financially cost-effective for HCPs to spend the time with patients to develop the sort of substantive relationships that allow for a deeper understanding of patients and their conditions.[15] Thus, while sometimes HCPs will have no recourse other than simply to comply with patients' health care decisions, greater expectations are not unreasonable. Moreover, I have tried to show that being sensitive to the dynamics of a situation is in fact part and parcel of the process of respecting patients' autonomous decisions, and that not to be concerned with what lies behind a patient's decision is to fail to take seriously respecting her autonomy. If Leo's dominant and underlying concern was his desire to feel empowered in some way, then were Shaun to miss that dynamic Shaun would be misunderstanding the very nature and meaning of Leo's decision. This is not to say that barriers to genuine communication, much less barriers to achieving consensus regarding the appropriate course of action, will not exist. But to think that respecting Leo's exercise of autonomy involves nothing more than simple acquiescence to the face value of his decisions is at best negligent and at worst malicious.

Another barrier to respecting patients' autonomy that is often particularly obstructive and pervasive concerns institutional structure. Take the previously mentioned hospital scenario wherein staffing patterns and policies regarding physician-nurse conduct actually precipitated conflicts with patients' autonomous decisions. Such examples illustrate that overattention to individual conflicts involving the exercise of autonomy sometimes can actually obscure the underlying barriers to realizing respect for autonomy—here, the lack of communication (about patient care) between nurses and physicians and perhaps the problematic nature of current medical hierarchy. Hence, an additional and important qualification to the model I have presented is that we not assume that just because "respect for patients' autonomy" frames an ethical conflict the only relevant ethical concerns are those that focus on the immediate conflict.

A perhaps more complicated issue is the specific responsibilities that attend particular relationships. I already have suggested that as more or less full-bodied enterprises patient-HCP encounters will depend upon the nature and dynamics of the existing relationship. So, that Shaun has known Leo for two years and has built up a friendship and sense of trust presumably gives Shaun access to a deeper level of communication and intimacy than might otherwise be the case.[16] An equally important influence on the nature of such interactions, however, is the the way in which *professional* responsibilities play a role in defining the patient-HCP relationship. Health care providers, for example, have duties to provide comparable service to all patients, not violate the law, refrain from making sexual advances on patients, and report the occurrence of certain infectious diseases. Of particular importance for the principle of respect for autonomy, however, are those professional responsibilities that focus on the *goals* of medicine and more specifically the goals of the patient-HCP relationship. Generally speaking, HCPs are expected to work to at least maintain if not improve the health of their patients. In that sense, HCPs have a responsibility to do what is necessary (and reasonable)[17] to create the kind of relationship that will conduce to their patients' health. But part of this involves making judgments about what is and what is not involved in providing (good) health care, judgments that invariably will run counter to certain patient decisions and requests. In terms of respecting autonomy, then, the big question is, Which of these decisions and requests may HCPs legitimately decline? This is not an easy question to answer. HCPs have certain professional responsibilities to promote health, or at least do no harm, and these in part *define* their relationships with their patients. And yet I have argued throughout that HCPs also have ethical responsibilities to respect patients' autonomous PSR decisions.

It is worth noting, of course, that (much as some HCPs would like to think otherwise) professional codes of conduct are not sacred, they *do* change. Due in part to challenges from patients, a growing skepticism of paternalism, as well as an extension of our ethical traditions regarding rights to noninterference, HCPs do *not* have a professional responsibility to force unwanted intervention on autonomous patients.[18] What yet remains fuzzy, however, is the extent to which denying *requested but nonrecommended treatment* can be justified on the grounds of "professional responsibility." This fuzziness stems in part from disagreement over the availability of alternative access to health care. For to the extent that Western society's strict regulation of medical practitioners and medical practice has created a closed shop, a virtual monopoly on health care, HCPs, by virtue of their privileged status, may well have an obligation to provide requested treatment that otherwise might be available but is not. Perhaps more importantly, however, the fuzziness regarding HCPs' obligation to dispense treatment stems from ambiguity over when it is reasonable to expect HCPs to accede to patients' autonomous health care judgments.[19]

To be honest, I am not really sure how to deal with this. On the one hand, the arguments against paternalistic actions by HCPs seem most stably grounded in a patient's right to noninterference. And yet on the other hand, unless a patient's right to exercise her autonomy in PSR matters involves some claim rights against HCPs' paternalistic denials of treatment, respect for autonomous PSR decisions may enjoy a very limited application. Consider the case of Tanya, a twenty-two year old who is pregnant for the first time. Tanya has an active case of genital herpes one week prior to her due date and so is discussing the situation with her physician, Dr. Benée Fitzhugh. Because of the risk of infection during passage through the birth canal and the dire consequences that can befall a neonate infected with herpes simplex virus, the two agree that Benée will perform a cesarian section when Tanya goes into labor. But when Tanya requests that her tubes be tied after the baby has been delivered, Benée explains that she refuses such requests to all first-time mothers because she does not think it is in their best interest to close down the option of future pregnancy. Despite extended and conscientious discussion as well as Benée's admission that carrying out Tanya's request would involve virtually no additional medical risk, the two simply cannot agree. If my argument for the primacy of respecting autonomous PSR decisions cannot cover Tanya's situation, I am troubled. And yet it truly opens up a Pandora's box to suggest that having the right to exercise one's autonomy in PSR matters in and of itself creates specific claim rights to aid.

Though I will do no more than mention it, one possible approach for addressing such situations resembles Henry Shue's argument for basic rights, which would establish various guarantees of assistance for the exercise of autonomy in PSR matters. In brief, Shue's argument is that because the possession and exercise of certain rights are fundamental to having self-respect, we in society have a responsibility not just to avoid depriving individuals of such rights but to provide protection and, if necessary, aid to guarantee individuals the opportunity to exercise these rights. Applied to respect for autonomy, the basic idea is that if a patient's right to exercise her autonomy in PSR matters is to be genuine and meaningful, society must guarantee her the ability to exercise that right, which in the present context would involve guaranteeing certain health care services.[20] This said, the conflict between *autonomous requests for treatment* and *HCPs' decisions and professional responsibilities to provide only "appropriate treatment"* poses an important challenge for my position, and as such will require some qualification of what it means to respect patients' autonomous PSR decisions.

Conclusion

I have tried to provide a meaningful and realistic understanding of what it means to respect autonomous PSR decisions within the context of health care. Arguing that genuine understanding is fundamental to the project of respecting a patient's autonomous decisions, and often is more elusive than it might appear, I have tried to show that communication in the form of a dialogical process can contribute greatly to respecting autonomy. I have suggested that patient-HCP encounters constitute relationships and that dialogue provides a developmental, and in that sense educational, avenue for establishing interconnections between individuals and with the world at large. I have tried to explain that this potential for overcoming otherness and developing a deeper understanding of the meaning and nature of beliefs, practices, and values can have important practical benefits for the provision of health care as well as the process of respecting patients' exercise of autonomy.

Starting from the principlist position that patients' autonomous decisions should have primacy in PSR matters, I have argued that what is involved in respecting autonomy depends on both the circumstances of the situation and the dynamics of the relationships involved. I have tried to make clear that the principle of respect for autonomous PSR decisions is not a totalizing theory but rather a side constraint. For not all bioethics conflicts will focus on the issue of respect for autonomy, nor should acting out of respect for autonomy be regarded as the only appropriate motivation for HCPs. Moreover, I have acknowledged that in a number of respects HCPs' actual responsibilities in terms of respecting patients' autonomy are indeterminate, and that resolutions to conflicts may require significant negotiation. In this respect I have tried to show that dialogue has distinct advantages over other ways of dealing with conflict both because dialogue is adaptable, and hence able to accommodate most any concern that is raised, and because it is an educational, enriching process in its own right. I have tried to convey that the medical environment provides a particularly lively stage for the playing out of conflicts involving autonomy, not only due to the vitality of the situations that arise within medicine, but also due to medicine's long tradition of paternalism and unequal power relations. There are questions that remain unanswered, but I hope to have shown that it is possible to stand firm by the principle of respect for patients' exercise of autonomy in PSR matters without denying the importance of relationships or ignoring the realities of medical practice.

What follows is a final dialogue that addresses many of the individual, relational, and institutional issues raised with regard to respecting patients' autonomous PSR decisions. The scenario itself is as common as it is complex. As with the previous dialogues, it is based on an actual clinical experience; hence many of the issues are nuanced rather than neon, and characters reflect the imperfections found in us all. As a model, this dialogue is meant to convey that attention to process, not adherence to strict principles, characterizes respect for autonomy. Relationships frame and define the boundaries within which the process of respecting autonomy takes place, and yet the focus remains on the individual, as it should. For respecting autonomy is an irreducibly individual matter on both ends of the equation.

Dialogue 5: Restraint by Any Other Name

Margaret Rose is eighty-four years old and now lives in a nursing home that most people just call *County*. County is a moderately large nursing home that provides independent care, intermediate care, and skilled care to roughly equivalent segments of its population. Of County's 240 residents, the vast majority (approximately 200) are female and about one-third are African-American or Latino/Latina. Almost 90 percent have some physical or mental impairment, and more than half are supported by Medicare or another form of public aid.

County is one of the better nursing homes in the area but is still plagued by the problems that confront most long-term care facilities: underfunding, inadequate facilities, relative isolation from its base community, high staff turnover, and, perhaps most acutely, understaffing. On average there are just over 3 registered nurses (RNs) and another 4 licensed practical nurses (LPNs) for every 100 residents. But since each resident is present twenty-four hours a day, seven days a week, while a full-time employee works, on average, thirty-three hours a week, the numbers are more like 1.5 licensed nursing personnel per 100 residents.[21] Further, licensed nurses spend most of their time filling out paperwork or handing out medicines. So hands-on care is relegated to certified nursing assistants (CNAs), who typically have less than a month of training, often have not completed high school, and get paid about $6.50 an hour for work that is extremely demanding and frequently unpleasant. As it turns out, more than 90 percent of County's residents need help bathing, about 75 percent need help dressing, 60 percent cannot go to the toilet by themselves or get to all the places they need to without assistance, and almost 30 percent need some help eating.

Margaret Rose has lived at County for about eight months. She had lived independently for four years after her husband, John, died. But last winter Margaret fell and broke her hip. After getting out of the hospital Margaret's daughter, Maureen Mayer, convinced Margaret to give County's independent care living arrangement a try. Shortly after moving to County, however, Margaret contracted pneumonia. After a short stay in the hospital and a somewhat prolonged recovery, Margaret is back to her old self, but weaker than before. Because of this weakened state and the fact that later in the spring she fell and hurt herself twice, Margaret was moved to intermediate care one month ago. These days Margaret is alert and oriented, but getting a little forgetful. Worried that she will fall and injure herself again, the nurses at County have asked Margaret to call them when she wants to go somewhere. But despite her promises, Margaret has continued to walk unsupervised. The nurses have suggested that Margaret wear a "seat belt" to remind her to call the nurses when she wants to get up. But because the belt would not allow her to get up unaided, Margaret has repeatedly objected. Margaret's roommate, Ruth, has many of the same physical debilities as Margaret. Unlike Margaret, however, Ruth is in the beginning stages of senile dementia and is now regularly restrained in a wheelchair.

Like most rooms at County, Margaret and Ruth's room is 11 feet × 11 feet with two hospital beds, two small night tables with reading lamps, one large dresser with four drawers, one closet with a folding door, a window, and a small bathroom with a toilet, sink, and shower. A light-yellow curtain hangs along a center ceiling track and can be pulled to veil the far bed. Margaret has brought with her a small portable TV, various knickknacks, photos, and even a few plants. Margaret is speaking with Linnea, one of the CNAs, as Ruth, who is strapped into a wheelchair, looks on.

MARGARET: I'm old enough to be your grandmother and I'm telling you that I don't want one. So you can just *shoo*. (*Margaret waves Linnea away with the back of her hand.*)

LINNEA: (*wryly and looking at Margaret as if Margaret is being naughty*) Sometimes I swear you *are* my grandmother. But really . . . Margaret, I'm not going to force you. But if you fall again, I'm telling one of the nurses and they're going to make you to wear one, you hear? (*Linnea walks out.*)

RUTH: I like Linnea. She takes the time to talk to you. Not like some of the others.

MARGARET: (*stubbornly*) I am *not* going to wear one of those seat belts. I won't!

RUTH: I think she's real pretty. Some of the girls here are so fat. I think they steal our food and eat it. I came back last night and those Oreo cookies I had were all gone. They come in and take it when we're not here.

MARGARET: Huh? What are you talking about?

RUTH: I'm saying they're fat because they steal my food. One time I had some Halloween candy and after they cleaned the room all of it was gone—and there was a lot.

(*A grey-haired woman in lavender polyester pants and purple slippers shuffles past their open door half-grunting, half-humming to herself "mmh, mmh, mmh, mmh, mmh."*)

MARGARET: (*commenting on the woman who has just passed*) They let Mrs. Strawson walk wherever *she* wants. That's because that way they don't have to take care of her.

RUTH: I caught her stealing my food once, too. I yelled at her and she never came back. They said she was looking for her husband and not to yell at her. But why was she trying to take my food? It's *my* food!

MARGARET: I don't care what they say. I'm going for a walk. Do you want to go to the TV room and watch a talk show?

(*Ruth nods and follows Margaret out of the room, using her feet to propel her wheelchair. The hallway is long and would be quite spacious were it not for the people parked along the walls. To use the handrails attached to the walls Margaret would have to navigate around the residents anchored in their wheelchairs and geri-chairs. So instead Margaret makes her way down the center of the hall, periodically reaching out to steady herself on the human pedestals she passes. Margaret and Ruth make their way down to the main hallway, which is kept clear, and then to the residents' lounge, where they join five or six other women already watching TV. An additional three residents sit in the corner of the lounge strapped to their wheelchairs, not interacting, apparently "vegged out." Just before entering the residents' lounge Margaret passes the staff lounge, where Linnea is sitting talking with another CNA, Laura. Diane Biggs, the head charge nurse at County, is also in the staff lounge doing some paperwork. County's administrative director of nursing is Beverly Katz, but Diane Biggs actually oversees nursing activity on the floor.*)

LINNEA: (*shouting to Margaret as she passes*) Be careful, now! We don't want you falling. Give us a call when you're ready to go back. OK?

(*Margaret keeps going and does not respond. She is beyond earshot, but just barely, when the women begin to talk about her.*)

LAURA: Old bitch! What a pain in the ass. Always has to be different.

LINNEA: She does push it, that's for sure. She tells me she used to teach school—you can tell she's used to being in charge. Ya gotta give her credit, though—she's a pistol.

LAURA: Maybe. But she's trouble. If she falls and hurts herself it's gonna be our ass, not hers, that's in hot water. And the way she acts . . . like this is some hotel and she's paying for private service. Get a life! Can you imagine what it'd be like if everyone expected to be treated like that? They'd be doin' whatever they wanted like there was no tomorrow.

DIANE: (*looking up from her work*) Have you talked to her daughter? She's a real nice lady.

LINNEA: You mean Maureen?

DIANE: Uh-huh. She comes in every Saturday, rain or shine.

LAURA: Well, somebody better get to talkin' to Moh-reeeen about her mother. That woman needs to learn that this ain't no resort. We got rules here . . .

(*The three women hear a clatter. Laura gets up and looks out the door of the staff lounge and into the residents' lounge. She sees Margaret in a heap in front of the TV with a folding tray table and a deck of playing cards on the floor.*)

LAURA: (*to Linnea and Diane*) See, what'd I tell ya? It's that woman's own damn fault if she broke her hip. Let's go see what she did to herself—like we ain't got better things to be doin'.

(*The three women move to where Margaret has now propped herself up on the floor. The TV is still blaring. Two of the residents are standing looking down at Margaret, one is at the door of the lounge where she had gone to go get help, while the others continue to watch TV. The three residents in the corner of the room in geri-chairs do not seem to have noticed that Margaret has fallen. One of them is drooling on a blue and white striped T-shirt, the other two appear to be staring off into space.*)

LINNEA: (*soothingly, as one would speak to a child*) Margaret, are you OK?

MARGARET: (*impatiently*) I just need to stand up. I'm fine.

DIANE: Do you hurt anywhere, Margaret?

MARGARET: Of course I hurt. I just fell didn't I?

LAURA: If you hadn't been walkin' around you'd've been fine. Ya see what you get for actin' like you do? You oughta do like Ruth here. You get around fine in that wheelchair, don't ya, Ruth?

RUTH: (*very cheerily*) Oh yeah, I get around fine.

DIANE: Which side did you fall on, Margaret?

MARGARET: On my backside. I'm fine. I just need to get up.

DIANE: OK. Let's just try and do it nice and slow. Linnea and I will help you.

(*Linnea and Diane lift Margaret and help her to her feet. She is a little wobbly, but she manages to steady herself after about fifteen seconds. As they work*) *on this Laura picks up the tray table and playing cards, muttering to herself as she puts the cards back in a stack on top of the TV.*)

LINNEA: Now, let's find you a place to sit . . . is this one OK? (*Somewhat embarrassed and wanting to be rid of all this attention, Margaret allows herself to be helped into the chair.*) Now I don't want you to try to get up without help, you hear?

LAURA: (*as she turns to leave*) You're lucky you didn't break your hip. (*muttering as she leaves*) No one but yourself to blame.

(*Diane watches as Linnea gets Margaret to agree to ask for help before trying to walk back to her room. Diane and Linnea leave the room together.*)

DIANE: It's not going to work, is it?

LINNEA: I don't think so. She says she'll call for me, but I know she won't. She's stubborn as all get out.

DIANE: I think we need to talk to Margaret's daughter. I'll give her a call now and see if I can't arrange for her to stop in before she visits with her mother. I'll also try to reach Dr. Page to get a PRN[22] restraint order for the weekend.

(*A few hours later, after already arranging with Margaret's daughter, Maureen, to meet on Saturday, Diane speaks with Dr. Matthew Page by telephone.*)

DIANE: Hello Dr. Page, thanks for calling me back.

MATTHEW: That's no trouble, Diane. What can I do for you?

DIANE: It's Mrs. Rose—you know, the eighty-four-year-old woman who got pneumonia a few months back and has chronic hip trouble. She's having trouble walking and . . . well, we think she's going to need to be restrained. Can you authorize a posey vest, PRN?

MATTHEW: Sure, that's no problem . . . actually, isn't she the schoolteacher, sort of fiery?

DIANE: That's Margaret alright.

MATTHEW: Has she agreed to being restrained?

DIANE: Not yet. I've set up an appointment to talk with her daughter tomorrow about it and I'm hoping that she'll be able to convince her mother. But Margaret's already fallen three-four times in the last month and it's just been luck that she hasn't broken her hip again.

MATTHEW: Well, good luck. I'll be out there Monday afternoon if you have any problems. Just let my nurse know and I'll try to set aside some time.

DIANE: Thanks again, Dr. Page.

(*The next morning is Saturday and Maureen stops in at Diane's office.*)

DIANE: Good morning Mrs. Mayer. It's nice to see you again.

MAUREEN: You too. And please call me Maureen. Everyone else does.

DIANE: Have you seen your mother yet?

MAUREEN: Not yet. (*a little puzzled*) You wanted me to stop in first, didn't you?

DIANE: Of course. I'm sorry. I get so used to asking people that question, I forget . . . well, anyway, would you like some coffee?

MAUREEN: No thanks. I just had breakfast. (*she pauses and then inquires with a bit of apprehension*) Is everything alright with Mother? I just spoke with her last night.

DIANE: Your mother's just fine. It's just that, well, we're starting to get concerned about her walking. She's not that steady anymore and we're worried she's going to fall and break something. Did she tell you that she fell again yesterday afternoon?

MAUREEN: (*surprised and a little alarmed*) No. No, she didn't. Is she alright? She didn't hurt her hip again, did she? (*shaking her head, Maureen says to herself under her breath*) That woman is so *stubborn*.

DIANE: No. She's alright for now. But that's exactly what we're concerned about. We're afraid she's going to fall and break something, maybe even wind up back in the hospital. And frankly, that's why I wanted to speak with you. Your mother doesn't . . . well, she isn't always the most cooperative. We've asked her to call us when she wants to go somewhere. But she's so independent, she just does what she wants. (*Diane pauses for a few moments, then continues a little hesitantly.*) We really don't think she ought to be walking unassisted. (*she hesitates*) We think she needs to be restrained.

(*Diane watches Maureen for her reaction. Maureen does not respond immediately. Instead, she purses her lips, wrinkles her forehead, and sighs as she lets out a deep breath.*)

MAUREEN: (*clearly disconcerted*) Have you talked to my mother about this?

DIANE: Not yet. But I think she knows it's coming. And I don't need to tell you that she's not going to like this, not one little bit. But if we don't do something . . .

MAUREEN: (*sighing again*) I understand. Uh . . . mmh . . . Is there any other alternative? My father's sister had Alzheimer's and had to be restrained. Every time we went to visit I remember my mother used to say how she'd never want to be like that, how terrible it must be to be tied up . . . it's just that my mother's so used to being independent that . . . (*Maureen's voice trails off as she loses herself in thought.*)

DIANE: I understand. Nobody prepares us for this sort of thing. Society doesn't want to think about it. Even the independent care residents *right here at County* don't want to think about it. As many people as are getting old . . . you'd think someone would be concerned enough to help us avoid using them. But until buildings get designed differently or somehow the patient load decreases, we just don't have the time or resources we need. I mean, I've got one girl today taking care of fourteen residents!

MAUREEN: (*Maureen waits, then responds*) So, you'd like me to talk with my mother about this?

DIANE: Yes. I'm sorry, I sort of got carried away there for a minute. We deal with this issue all the time, and sometimes I just wish . . . well anyway, that's my problem, not yours. But I would appreciate it if you would speak with your mother and help her understand that she really does need to be restrained . . . for her own good.

MAUREEN: (*joking*) You sure you wouldn't rather have this pleasure?

(*Diane smiles back and the two women, each in their midfifties, stand up and shake hands. As Maureen turns to leave, Diane gives her a kind and empathetic look.*)

DIANE: I know this is hard. Why don't you stop in before you leave? If I'm not here, just have the receptionist page me. Good luck.

(*Maureen walks down the hall toward her mother's room. It's about 10:15 A.M. Normally, Maureen arrives around 10:00 after Margaret has had her breakfast and returned to her room. In the past the two would sit and talk, often go out shopping if Margaret was feeling up to it, have a late lunch or early dinner at some restaurant, and come back in the late afternoon. Maureen enjoys spending time with Margaret. But as her mother has become increasingly weak it is Maureen's sense of filial duty as much as anything that motivates her weekly visits. When Maureen arrives at her mother's room, Margaret and Ruth are playing dominoes. Though Margaret always wins at dominoes, she often helps Ruth earn a better score. The two women have lived together for a month and get along very nicely, especially for people who had never known each other before.*)

MAUREEN: Good morning Mother! Hello Ruth! Who's winning today? (*Margaret gives her daughter a knowing look. Maureen in turn moves over to look at the score and squeezes her mother's hand.*) Looks like you're giving my mother a run for her money today, Ruth.

(*Ruth smiles at Maureen and then places a domino down. She looks up again and smiles broadly.*)

MAUREEN: Is it OK if I take my mother away from you? I think we're going to go out for a while. (*Still holding Margaret's hand, Maureen turns to her mother.*) Are you up for that?

MARGARET: I sure am. (*smiling*) You're saving me from Ruth, don't you know.

(*Maureen helps Margaret up out of her chair and into a light blue sweater that matches the wall of her room. Maureen takes her mother's arm and as they start down the hall, she pays special attention to her mother's gait and tries to keep her steady.*)

MARGARET: (*a little petulantly*) I can walk, you know.

MAUREEN: I know. I'm just trying to help. *You're* a little touchy this morning.

MARGARET: (*still a bit petulant*) Everyone seems to think I'm not capable of getting myself around anymore. I haven't needed anyone's help walking for better than eighty-two years and I don't see any reason to start now.

MAUREEN: (*showing deference to her mother, but challenging her nonetheless*) They told me you fell yesterday.

MARGARET: (*sarcastically*) Oh they did, did they? Well, they should mind their own business. And if there weren't so many things in your way around here, it'd be easier for a person to move around, anyhow.

MAUREEN: Don't you think you're being a little critical, Mother? Compared to a lot of other places they do a very nice job here. Everyone I've met has been friendly and very helpful. You were just telling me the other day how one of the aides helped you sew a button.

MARGARET: It depends who you get. Some of 'em would just as soon trip you as help you up. See that one over there, Laura's her name? I think she rides a broom at night.

MAUREEN: *Mother!!*

MARGARET: I'm telling you, all that one there wants to do is smoke her cigarettes and gab. And the more of us get out of their way, the less work they have to do. (*Maureen looks at her mother as if it is clear that Margaret is exaggerating.*) You don't believe me? You just stay here and watch sometime—you get tied down (*practically spitting out her disgust*) . . . peh! . . . you're as good as forgotten.

MAUREEN: Mother, that's not true. These are nice people doing the best they can.

MARGARET: Well, it's not very good.

MAUREEN: Mother, I don't think you're being fair. Sometimes people have to be restrained for their own good.

MARGARET: As far as I can tell, once they get you so you can't move around like you want, you might as well pack it up. I've seen 'em. People go downhill so fast you'd think they fell off a cliff. First they tie you down, next thing you know you're in a corner drooling on your bathrobe.

MAUREEN: Mother, you act like this is some conspiracy. This is a nursing home for God's sake. It's set up to help people who need help taking care of themselves. When you came in here you understood this wasn't a resort. They have their own rules and by deciding to live here you agreed to abide by them. They have over two hundred people living here and they simply don't have time to be watching out for you constantly. If you weren't so stubborn and always having to do everything your own way, you'd make it a lot easier on yourself, you know. You have to learn to compromise.

MARGARET: That's easy for you to say. No one's trying to tie you down.

MAUREEN: Mother, you're going to get hurt. We're not even out of the building yet and twice now I've kept you from stumbling. You have to be realistic.

MARGARET: (*indignantly*) I know what I'm capable of. I don't need anybody telling me what I can and can't do. Why, in my classroom . . .

MAUREEN: (*more gently*) Mom, you're not in your class now. You're in a nursing home.

MARGARET: (*refusing to concede her position*) You make it sound like I chose to come here of my own free will. Well, I didn't. It wasn't like I had much choice! (*her voice has become a mixture of anger and pouting*) You don't understand what it's like to be old. Everybody leaves, you have to fend for yourself, and then when you can't make it on your own anymore they put you out here and tell you you agreed to it. Well, I didn't. I didn't agree to it at all. And if it takes making people angry to keep what I have left, then that's the way it's going to be. If I'm gonna hurt myself, then that's my business as far as I'm concerned. Nobody's gonna tie me down!

MAUREEN: (*As they walk across the parking lot, Maureen begins to recognize that this is a much deeper issue than she initially had thought.*) Mom, what happens when you talk to the nurses about it? Do they understand how you feel about this?

MARGARET: (*shaking her head*) Mo, you just don't understand. Nobody ever talks to us.

MAUREEN: Mother, that's not true. I've seen you with that girl, what's her name, Linnea. And they talk to you when they do music and games. And what about when you made that lovely needlepoint pillow for me and Fred? You told me yourself how they helped you.

MARGARET: That's not what I'm talking about. Sure, they do those things. But when it comes to how they're going to treat you, you can forget it. Nobody asks you where you want to live. You can't even leave the dining room when you want to. What makes you think anyone's going to ask me whether I want to be tied down? They're not stupid. No one in their right mind *wants* to be tied down. Why, I bet you right now they've got some plan for trying to tie me down. Probably asked you to talk me into it, didn't they?

MAUREEN: (*feeling a little guilty, if not naive*) Well . . . they did ask me to talk about it with you. But Mother, they're worried about you. What if you fall? Have you thought about that? You'd be back in the hospital . . . you *are* eighty-four, you know. I don't think you're being realistic. If you make too much trouble, they might not even let you back in. (*Maureen helps her mother into the car.*) Look, you wait here. I need to go in and talk to the nurse for a minute. I'm gonna see if we can all get together and work this thing out. I can take an afternoon off from work next week. OK? (*Maureen waits for a response, but all she gets is a sarcastic look.*) Have it your way. I'll be back in a minute. Oh, I brought you an Andrews Sisters tape. It's in the tape deck now—here are the keys . . . I'll be back soon.

MARGARET: (*as Maureen goes back into the nursing home, Margaret says to herself*) I'll walk when I *wanna* walk!

MAUREEN: (*seeing Diane in the hall*) Oh, Mrs. Biggs!

DIANE: Hi again. Oh, and please, call me Diane.

MAUREEN: OK, Diane. Well, I tried talking to my mother and . . . she's being very difficult about this. Will you be here this afternoon when we get back, say, around 5:00?

DIANE: I'm afraid not. I leave at 1:00 on Saturdays. I'm in all next week, though. In fact, Dr. Page said he'd be in on Monday. Maybe the three of us could get together and try to work this out. I really think it's something that we need to get settled.

MAUREEN: Monday would be wonderful. Could we do it late afternoon, say, around 4:00?

DIANE: That would be fine.

MAUREEN: Will that woman, Linnea, the aide who takes care of Mother, be around then? I get the feeling she might be able to help us figure out how best to work this.

DIANE: Uh . . . we don't normally include CNAs in planning meetings.

Um . . . that's not to say that we can't, but normally they're so busy and they're not . . . well, um, I'll see if she's working. (*more to herself than to Maureen*) She normally does days—which means she gets off at 3:30. Uh, well, let me see what I can do.

MAUREEN: I'd really appreciate that. Mother is just . . . well, particular, if you know what I mean. And she really has a thing about being independent. (*remembering her mother's comment*) You weren't planning on making her use a wheelchair or anything like that this weekend were you? 'Cause I think that would really upset her.

DIANE: Actually, I did phone Dr. Page for a PRN restraint order. But if you feel strongly about it I'm sure we can hold off until next week. You do realize, though, that your mother is at risk for falling and hurting herself. And at her age it could be quite serious.

MAUREEN: (*nodding her head with resignation*) I understand. But let's at least wait 'til Monday. I don't think she'd forgive me if I let her be tied down.

DIANE: (*All too familiar with this situation, Diane nods in assent.*) OK. Just so you understand the situation. Monday at 4:00, then. Have a nice time with your mother.

MAUREEN: Bye-bye.

(*The rest of the day is uneventful for Margaret and Maureen. They go shopping, have a pleasant early dinner, and return to County around 5:30. Maureen explains that she and Diane have arranged a meeting for Monday afternoon and that no one will interfere with Margaret between now and then. The next morning, however, Margaret falls on the way to lunch while trying to go around two residents in wheelchairs who had stopped to talk. Luckily, Margaret's only injury is a skin tear on her right elbow. About 3:30 Monday afternoon Maureen arrives at County, checks in with Diane, and then goes down to her mother's room. Margaret is a little anxious about what will happen at today's meeting.*)

MARGARET: What do you mean I'm not supposed to come to the meeting!?!

MAUREEN: Just not at first.

MARGARET: (*rather upset*) What do you all have to say that I can't hear?! I pay my taxes. I have the same rights as anyone else. *I'm* the one that lives here, you know!

MAUREEN: I know, Mother. They just want to talk it over with Dr. Page and . . . look, I don't know why you're not supposed to be there at first. But that's the way they want it. Why do you always have to fight everything? They probably just want to make sure that everyone understands the situation.

MARGARET: If that's all they want to do, then why can't I be there?

MAUREEN: (*exasperated and having no real answer*) I don't *know*, Mother! Can't you just let it be? I'm told that, usually, residents don't even participate in these kinds of meetings. And they even made a special effort to have that aide you like there. If you're too demanding, people'll stop listening.

MARGARET: I don't think they listen at all.

MAUREEN: Mother, that's not fair and you know it. Now, stop.

MARGARET: (*pouting*) This whole thing isn't fair.

MAUREEN: No one said the world was totally fair. Everyone's doing the best they can. You just need to be a little more tolerant, that's all.

MARGARET: I don't *want* to be more tolerant. I'm not a child and this is a decision that's mine to make. If I want to walk around and fall down that's my business.

MAUREEN: It is *not* just *your* business. These people are here to take care of you and you can't just ignore everything around you. You're in a nursing home, Mother! (*She sighs and tries to regain the calm she had just a few minutes before.*) I'm not going to argue with you about this. In a few minutes we're going to walk down to Mrs. Biggs's office and you're going to have to wait until they're ready for you to join us. That's just the way it is . . .

MARGARET: (*under her breath, but loud enough for her daughter to hear*) It may be the way it is, but it certainly doesn't *have* to be that way.

MAUREEN: That may be so. But there's nothing we can do to change the situation now. So let's just make the best of it, alright? (*She waits, without getting a response.*) Alright?!

MARGARET: (*her voice thick with sarcasm*) Whatever you say.

MAUREEN: (*exasperated, but no longer reacting argumentatively*) Mother, what am I going to do with you?

MARGARET: You don't *have* to do anything!

MAUREEN: (*Taking a deep breath, Maureen opens her bag and removes a small Tupperware container.*) Here, the girls baked you some cookies yesterday—your favorite, poppy seed.

MARGARET: (Margaret accepts the peace offering graciously.) What a lovely present! (*then, gently mockingly*) It's a shame their mother doesn't have as much respect for *her* elders.

MAUREEN: (*shaking her head, and with good-humored frustration*) *You* are terrible.

(*As Maureen and her mother enter Diane's office they are greeted by Diane.*)

DIANE: Hi there Margaret, Maureen. We're going to meet down in Beverly Katz's office. Dr. Page is already down there, and Linnea's supposed to meet us there in a few minutes.

(*The three women walk two doors down the hall. They enter a room where a secretary is typing. The secretary stops momentarily and tells them to please go right in.*)

DIANE: Margaret, why don't you just take a seat over there. We'll come out and get you in a little bit. OK?

MARGARET: No, that's not OK. I don't see why . . .

MAUREEN: (*Somewhat embarrassed, Maureen turns to Margaret and speaks with a sternness in her voice.*) Mother, we talked about this. Now, we'll be out in just a little bit. Please be patient. There are some nice magazines right over there.

(*Reluctantly, Margaret goes over to an orange-brown couch along the wall and after picking out a month-old copy of* Newsweek *from the endtable seats herself on the couch. As Maureen follows Diane into the inner office both Nurse Beverly Katz and Dr. Matthew Page rise, leaving off their conversation.*)

BEVERLY: It's so good to see you again, Mrs. Mayer. (*They shake hands. Then, gesturing toward Matthew*) I believe you've met Dr. Page before.

MAUREEN: Briefly, a couple of times, I think. (*Maureen extends her hand to Matthew and the two shake hands and smile politely at each other.*)

MATTHEW: (*His tone is warm, but very professional—almost stiff in contrast with Diane's and Beverly's.*) Yes, we met when your mother first came here and then sometime this spring, wasn't it?

MAUREEN: That's right. You had on that same blue blazer. (*Then, sensing her faux pas, Maureen starts to apologize.*) I mean . . .

MATTHEW: Oh, that's alright. A lot of people kid me about it. It's sort of gotten to be a habit with me. I trained up at Mayo and they always had us wear these, and I guess I just got used to it. Now I can't seem to feel at home practicing medicine without it.

BEVERLY: (*pleasantly but clearly meaning to be efficient*) Well, shall we get down to business? Diane, why don't you and Mrs. Mayer sit over there on the couch and I'll come around here. (*somewhat quizzically*) You say Linnea will be joining us too? (*Diane nods.*) That's fine. And Margaret's just outside, is that right? (*Again, Diane nods as everyone takes a seat.*) Good . . . now, as I understand it Margaret has been with us at County for about eight months but it's only about a month ago that she was moved from independent care to intermediate care. She came here because . . . (*Beverly leafs through the folder on her lap*) because of a broken hip that was surgically repaired . . . but it was decided that she needed more attention than the family could provide at home. Is that right?

MAUREEN: That's pretty much it. We have two girls in high school and two boys in junior high, and it gets pretty busy and crowded sometimes. It just didn't seem to be the best thing for Mother. She thought so herself.

BEVERLY: And now Diane tells me that Margaret's getting more unsteady on her feet. Diane, you say she's fallen a number of times recently?

DIANE: Mm-hm. She's fallen five times in the last two weeks, and those are just the ones we've seen. (*turning to Maureen*) I just found out she fell again yesterday morning on the way to lunch. (*As Maureen shakes her head, Diane turns back to Beverly and Matthew.*) Luckily, she hasn't hurt herself yet. But yesterday she did get a skin tear on her arm. And the staff is worried that she's going to break her hip again . . . or worse.

BEVERLY: So, the question is, What do we do?

DIANE: We've already asked her to call one of the aides when she wants to go somewhere. But even though she agrees, she almost never does. To be honest, even if she did call someone, there wouldn't always be an aide available. And given how strong-minded she is, I think she'd just get up and try to do it herself. (*Maureen nods.*) I don't see much alternative to restraining her. We can't just let Margaret put herself in danger like that.

MATTHEW: What's her mental status?

DIANE: She's definitely all there . . . and then some.

MATTHEW: And her view toward her situation?

DIANE: I guess that depends on who you ask. She's a very independent woman, a former schoolteacher. Some of the aides say she can get pretty unreasonable at times.

MATTHEW: Why's that?

DIANE: I guess . . . she just wants to do what she wants to do.

MAUREEN: I think she's afraid of losing her independence. (*As Maureen talks it is clear that she is both sympathetic and skeptical of her mother's views.*) She seems to think that if she allows herself to be restrained she'll get ignored and, as she puts it, wind up in the corner staring off into space and drooling on herself.

MATTHEW: (*Matthew rubs his brow with the fingers of his right hand.*) You have to admit, it's not a very attractive picture.

MAUREEN: But it's not true . . . is it?

MATTHEW: Well, studies show that as the elderly, or anyone for that matter, lose what they conceive of as their power to be independent they tend to deteriorate at a much more rapid pace than one would predict from their physiological state alone. There is no clearly established cause and effect, but it is nonetheless an observed correlation.

BEVERLY: It's certainly one of the difficulties we face as an institution. On the one hand, we'd like to make it possible to keep as many people out of restraints as we can, and yet to make the kinds of changes necessary to maintain a safe restraint-free environment . . . well, it's not going to happen any time soon.

MAUREEN: Mother does complain that all the wheelchairs in the hallways make its hard to get around.

BEVERLY: That's just one thing. In addition to the physical plant, there's the additional personnel we'd need to provide more individualized supervision, the additional time and support from physicians to thoroughly assess residents' drug regimens, mental status, as well as underlying medical condition. We really need to have more physical therapy. If the CNA turnover wasn't so high, residents would have better continuity of care . . . the list just goes on and on. I have a lot of sympathy for what Dr. Page is saying. But County, like most other nursing homes, simply doesn't have the resources to become restraint-free. What we'd really need is one-to-one supervision, and that's just not a reality.

MAUREEN: I see.

MATTHEW: Of course, not all of County's residents have the cognitive capacity that Mrs. Rose has. It sounds as if she's unsteady on her feet. But given what Mrs. Biggs says and what I recall from my last interaction with your mother, Mrs. Rose is perfectly competent to gauge her situation.

DIANE: That may be, but (*turning to Maureen momentarily*), with all due respect, she's not doing a very good job of it. And if she hurts herself she's going to be in a worse situation. Part of my job is to make sure that the people under my care don't get hurt, and I can't very well do that if people who shouldn't be up walking by themselves are out doing that.

BEVERLY: (*looking around the room*) Well, what are our alternatives here?

(*There is a knock on the door and Linnea peeks her head in. Beverly motions her to enter, which she does. Linnea clearly feels and is perceived of as out of place. She has never been included in a care-plan conference. She takes one of the two empty seats, places her bag next to her on the floor, and smooths her skirt as she puts her knees together.*)

BEVERLY: (*to Linnea*) We were just discussing how to deal with Margaret. The consensus seems to be that given the operations here at County and the increasing difficulties that Margaret is having walking, we're facing a potentially serious problem. And the question is, How do we deal with it? By the way, Dr. Page, this is Linnea; Linnea, Dr. Page. (*They nod to each other politely.*)

MATTHEW: Has anyone spoken with Mrs. Rose about this?

MAUREEN: I've tried to. My mother's just so stubborn, though.

MATTHEW: Linnea, are you the person who takes care of Mrs. Rose on a day-to-day basis?

LINNEA: (*Linnea speaks with some hesitation.*) Uh . . . yeah, pretty much. I work the 7:00 to 3:30 shift every day but Sunday. And, well . . . I usually get Margaret and Ruth, both, because I like 'em and 'cause Margaret can be pretty hard on ya, and some of the others don't like that much. (*After speaking, Linnea lowers her eyes.*)

MATTHEW: Linnea, in your estimation, what would you say is Mrs. Rose's mental status? (*Matthew notices that Linnea looks a little confused by the question.*) That is, would you say that Mrs. Rose is capable of making sound judgments?

LINNEA: She's real smart, if that's what you mean.

MATTHEW: Well, that's certainly part of it. But I'm also interested in whether you think that Mrs. Rose understands the nature of her condition and the risks she's taking.

LINNEA: (*smiling*) Oh, she understands everything, alright! That woman's sharp as a tack. She's even got Ruth, that's her roommate, tryin' to do more stuff for herself. Margaret sort of likes to take people under her wing. She was a schoolteacher, you know. Only I imagine she's more impatient with people now. But yeah, I'd say she's on top of things.

MATTHEW: Hm. (*There is moment or two of silence.*)

BEVERLY: (*very matter of fact*) It seems to me there are a couple of options. On the one hand we could place Margaret in limited restraints, most likely a wheelchair with a posey vest. That way she could get around but wouldn't be able to try to walk without assistance. This would compromise her independence somewhat but it also would protect her from incurring a serious injury. Alternatively, we could not impose any physical restrictions at all. Certainly this would preserve her independence. But it would allow Margaret to continue to jeopardize her health. In particular, it would be more likely that she might fall and perhaps compromise her subsequent capacity for independence. She hasn't been particularly cooperative, so I'm not sure how much of her assistance we can rely on for this decision. Does that seem right to you, Diane?

DIANE: That's been my experience. (*turning to Maureen*) One of the problems, as you can imagine, is that by acceding to residents' demands for independence we can wind up actually helping undermine their independence. They get to be like children in a way. They want what they want *now*, and they just don't think about the future. With a lot of the residents this isn't as much of a dilemma because their mental status is compromised and they really can't understand the risks. But with people like your mother it's . . . there's a real conflict because they have the capacity to make a good judgment but they're just not exercising it. So while we'd like to respect their wishes, it's really not in their best interest.

MAUREEN: I understand. And my mother can be so difficult. I'm sure you do the best you can here. I'm just worried that if she does lose some of her independence she'll stay angry and maybe lose her . . . I don't know . . . her sense of self, I guess. She's not used to being in a position where she doesn't have control.

BEVERLY: I know it sounds a little heartless. But sometimes it's a good thing for residents to be a little angry. It keeps them fighting. And at that age fighting is part of what living is about. As long as they're battling there's hope. (*Beverly pauses and watches Maureen, who seems uncomfortable but resigned to the prospect of her mother being subjected to restraints.*) What do you think, Dr. Page?

MATTHEW: Uh . . . I guess I'd like to hear from Mrs. Rose herself. It's not that I necessarily disagree with what's been said. But different cases are so variable. What's appropriate for one person is contraindicated for another. You all are obviously much more familiar with the day-to-day goings-on at a nursing home. But . . . depending on a resident's personality, I'm not at all sure that it's helpful to set up a situation where a person's daily existence depends upon their ability to, as you say, engage in battle. (*Matthew pauses and takes a long, drawn-out breath that he then lets escape, registering his uncertainty.*) For example, I'm not sure that Linnea here has either the time or energy to battle with Mrs. Rose. (*At this, Linnea smiles sheepishly.*) And perhaps not all the aides will show Mrs. Rose the same patience and care as Linnea if forced to battle with her. I do understand that it's fairly easy for me to be a critic in this kind of situation. But it's ultimately my signature that has to go on any order for restraints, and I feel it's important to be clear about what is and is not the appropriate course of action.

BEVERLY: Linnea, could you get Margaret? . . . thanks . . . and do help her negotiate the carpet—we don't want her to hurt herself.

(*Linnea gets up and goes to fetch Margaret from the outer office. As Linnea helps Margaret make her way in everyone remains very quiet until Margaret is seated.*)

BEVERLY: Hello Margaret. I believe you know everyone. Do you remember Dr. Page?

MATTHEW: Hello Mrs. Rose. It's good to see you again.

MARGARET: Hello. I remember you. You're the one who treated me when I had pneumonia.

MATTHEW: That's right. I trust you're doing better now.

MARGARET: I am except that they don't want to let me walk. They think I'm too old. (*Margaret looks over at her daughter and then at Diane before returning her gaze to Matthew. Believing that this is meant to be an interrogation, Margaret waits to be asked whatever questions the group has for her.*)

MATTHEW: So tell me, Mrs. Rose, do *you* think you're too old to be walking?

MARGARET: (*resolutely*) I can walk just fine.

MAUREEN: Mother, you've fallen five times in the last two weeks.

MARGARET: (*impatiently to Maureen*) No one's asking you. (*turning back to Matthew*) I do get a little unsteady sometimes, but if I had a cane I think I'd do just fine.

MATTHEW: Have you used a cane before, and has that helped?

MARGARET: No one's ever offered me one.

MATTHEW: Why's that, do you think?

MARGARET: I don't know. Ask them. They're the ones that want to tie me down.

MATTHEW: Mrs. Rose, I don't think anyone wants to tie you down. They just want to make sure that you don't hurt yourself.

MARGARET: They want to tie me to a wheelchair so I can't get up and do as I want.

MATTHEW: Would that be so bad?

MARGARET: How would you like to be tied to something that you can't get away from?

MATTHEW: Well, I guess that all depends. If I was concerned about my safety and that was the best way to make sure that I didn't hurt myself, then it probably wouldn't bother me too much. But I get the feeling that you don't feel that way.

MARGARET: No I don't. You don't know what it's like living here. They already take away everything you're used to. You can't even keep food in your room without them taking it.

DIANE: That's because of roaches, Margaret. You know that.

MARGARET: (*ignoring Diane's comment*) And I've seen what happens once they tie you down. You can't even go to the bathroom by yourself. (*look-*

ing over toward Linnea and then back at Matthew) They don't even have enough girls to get you to breakfast on time. You think they're going to be around if you need 'em and you can't get up? No sir.

MATTHEW: Hmph. That doesn't sound too good. But I understand that the aides *have* offered to help you walk, but that you don't call them.

MARGARET: I like to keep my business private. If I want to go somewhere, I don't see why everyone should have to know about it.

MATTHEW: Well, I guess the problem is, Mrs. Rose, that you might fall and hurt yourself if you walk without help. That's why everyone's so concerned.

MARGARET: Two women last week, Mrs. Bell and Mrs. Washington, you tell them about not getting hurt. They fell out of bed *because* somebody tied them to their bedrails and they tried to climb out to go to the bathroom. And just yesterday Mr. Murphy about choked trying to get out of the chair they tied him to. Linnea here cares, but some of the others I see tie people down just so they have less work. (*Unconsciously, Linnea nods in assent.*) I never even tied my dog up—I expect to be treated at least as good as that.

MAUREEN: (*to Matthew and Beverly*) You'll have to excuse my mother. She just gets upset about losing her independence. I know she thinks well of the people here—she tells me so.

MATTHEW: That's alright. We're here to find out what Mrs. Rose thinks and to see if we can't find a way to protect her values as well as her safety. (*turning back to Margaret*) Now, Mrs. Rose, I understand that you're worried about losing your independence here. And I'm beginning to realize that in addition to being an independent woman you're also a fairly private person. What I'd like to know from you is under what sorts of conditions you'd be willing to compromise some of your independence in order to . . .

MARGARET: I'm not willing to compromise *any* of my independence. That's about all I've got left. It may not look like much, but this is *my* life, not anybody else's.

MATTHEW: (*gently but still quite professionally*) Mrs. Rose, I'm not trying to take any of that away. I'm just trying to see if there isn't some way that we could work out an arrangement that allows you to be independent and yet recognizes the concerns that all of us have for your health. You've already said that a cane would help you. What would you think about an arrangement whereby, say, if you wanted to walk more than halfway down the hall, you'd call for some assistance and you'd agree to wait, let's say, ten minutes?

MARGARET: How do I know they'd come? I hear people calling for aides all the time and they don't come.

MATTHEW: Well, that would be part of the arrangement. If they didn't come within ten minutes, then you would just do it on your own. But this would be an agreement.

MARGARET: (*somewhat petulantly*) And what if I decided I didn't want to do that anymore?

MATTHEW: Well . . . that's what we're trying to work out.

MARGARET: What you're saying is if I don't agree they'll tie me down.

MAUREEN: Mother, that's not what we're saying. You're not listening to the doctor. He's trying to help and you're trying to find things to pick at. They can't have you walking around and falling all the time. It's too dangerous.

MARGARET: I wouldn't be hurting anyone but myself.

BEVERLY: Actually, Margaret, there is the matter of financial responsibility. Legally, we can be held liable for any physical demise we could reasonably have prevented. It's true enough that there aren't any definitive legal precedents, but as an institution we'd be putting ourselves at risk were you to fall and injure yourself.

DIANE: (*more to Matthew than Margaret*) You have to understand that as a long-term care institution part of what allows County to function is that we maintain certain policies that maximize residents' well-being while at the same time minimizing any disharmony. Because we're having to manage well over two hundred residents, there has to be some sort of consistency. And unfortunately sometimes that means that it's not possible to provide residents all the freedom they would otherwise have. It's sort of like having traffic laws.

MATTHEW: I understand what you're saying. But it seems to me that Margaret's situation isn't like driving in traffic. The only thing that's at stake here is her own well-being—assuming, of course, that litigation is not a factor. (*With this last comment, Matthew looks to Margaret expectantly.*)

MARGARET: I wouldn't sue anybody—as long as no one ties me down.

MAUREEN: (*in a tone that is at once sympathetic and resigned, Maureen almost declares to everyone in the room*) We're not suing anybody. (*then turning toward Margaret*) But Mother, you're not being reasonable here.

MARGARET: I don't have to be reasonable if I don't want to.

BEVERLY: Actually, Margaret, you did sign a contract agreeing to abide by the rules of this institution, and part of those rules include not deviating from the medical recommendations for your care. As a health care facility it wouldn't make sense for us to allow residents to engage in an activity that puts them at substantial risk.

MARGARET: (*Seeing this as a threat, Margaret begins to get a little scared. From looking at Beverly, she turns toward Matthew*) But you haven't said I needed to be restrained.

MATTHEW: That's right, I haven't. (*Seeing Margaret's fear, Matthew tries to reassure her.*) And at least for now let's assume that I won't. (*Matthew then looks around the room, making eye contact with each of the five women. Having gained more of a sense of calm in the room, Matthew then continues.*) Now as I understand it, we have a problem here. The problem is that Mrs. Rose, who everyone agrees is competent, is starting to have difficulty getting around on her own. (*now looking directly at Margaret*) The danger is that you will fall and hurt yourself. The nurses here at County are worried about that, as is your daughter. I think we all get the sense that you're very concerned that you not lose your sense of independence. And, perhaps justifiably, you even question whether restraints constitute an appropriate response—either because they are not that safe themselves or because they are used by the staff as a . . . how should I say . . . as a substitute for providing the sort of care that's actually warranted. On the other hand, Mrs. Katz is concerned that allowing you unrestricted mobility might jeopardize not only your own health but also the health of the larger institution, so to speak. Obviously, your daughter's concerns have to do with her desire to see that you are properly taken care of. The question, then, is how to resolve this impasse in a way that not only respects your wishes, Mrs. Rose, but also recognizes County's concerns and minimizes the chances of your encountering any disability. Does that seem to sum up the situation? (*Matthew looks around the room and, perceiving no dissent, arches his eyebrows and waits.*) So . . . ?

(*There is silence for some time.*)

DIANE: If you're asking me, I think Margaret's asking the nursing staff to condone her decision to disregard her own health. And I don't think that that's fair.

MARGARET: Well, I don't think that you have any business telling me what I should or shouldn't do. I'm not asking you to do anything more than what you're paid to do. And God knows I pay enough.

MAUREEN: Mother, please! We're trying to sort this out. You don't have to be antagonistic.

MARGARET: (*calming down a little*) Alright. Well let me put it this way, then. I don't see people getting better here. They get worse and worse and then they die. It seems to me that the least you can do is let a person get worse the way *they* want to get worse.

BEVERLY: I understand what you're saying, Margaret. But you have to realize that we can't just sit back and let people go downhill. It's our job to do as much as we can to preserve people's well-being.

MARGARET: If old people drooling in a corner is your idea of well-being . . . well, all I can say is that I never want to end up that way.

LINNEA: (*a little timidly, surprised at herself for speaking up*) But Margaret, you're not going to end up that way. Ruth maybe; but not you. It's your bones we're worried about. If you fall, you may never walk again. And then you'd be stuck in a wheelchair for sure.

(*This seems to strike a chord with Margaret. She does not respond. Sensing an inroad, Diane joins in.*)

DIANE: When people get to your age, women in particular, their bones get brittle. You've been fortunate so far. But another fall or two and you might not ever have a choice again. What we're trying to do is preserve your choices.

MARGARET: (*starting to feel defeated*) How do I know that? Some of the aides would keep me tied up all day—some of them have mean hearts. (*Linnea puts her hand on Margaret's arm.*)

MATTHEW: (*to Beverly and Diane*) What sorts of precautions are there for people in restraints? How often are they removed, for example? (*Beverly looks to Diane.*)

DIANE: Well, the guidelines say that they should be checked every half hour and that they should be removed once every hour so residents can move around a bit—so as not to get too stiff.

LINNEA: (*with a little more confidence*) But we don't really have time for all that. If I get to loosen someone's restraints twice a shift, that's really good. I usually have twelve patients, and at least six of them are in some kind of restraints. I just don't have time to untie them and exercise them—at least not if I'm going to finish all the other chores I have, like helping them get dressed and fed and changing the linen, not to mention transporting residents to activities. And the chances of my getting all that done depends a lot on whether everyone's being cooperative. (*stealing a glance at Margaret*) And not everyone always is.

MARGARET: (*to Matthew*) You see?

MATTHEW: I'm certainly starting to.

MARGARET: Who's to say I'll ever get out of them once they put me in restraints?

MAUREEN: Mother, don't you think you're being a little melodramatic here?

MARGARET: You want someone to tie you down? That's fine—I'm not stopping you. But that's not something I want to risk. (*to Beverly*) No offense, but I don't believe in giving anyone that kind of power over me.

(*Margaret's stubbornness hangs in the room and no one says anything for a few moments.*)

BEVERLY: (*taking a deep breath and then half-smiling*) Well . . . it sounds like at least we're clear on the different positions. I take it, Margaret, that you're not willing to accept any kind of restraint, even if it's just a posey vest, to remind you that you need help walking. (*Beverly looks inquisitively at Margaret, who lowers her chin, defiantly nodding her confirmation.*) And Diane, you feel that some form of restraint is warranted given Margaret's unsteadiness. Linnea, you too? (*Both Diane and Linnea nod their heads in agreement.*) Mrs. Mayer, what are your feelings here?

MAUREEN: I really don't know . . . I really want my mother to be safe. (*turning toward Margaret, but still talking to Beverly*) But I know how important it is for her to be independent. I think she's being unreasonable. But that's not really new. (*Maureen shakes her head.*) I just don't know.

BEVERLY: And you, Dr. Page?

MATTHEW: (*resuming a professional tone that again borders on being stiff*) Well, it seems to me that we're looking at a conflict between autonomy and beneficence here—or perhaps I should say paternalism. Medically speaking, it sounds as if Mrs. Rose is going to place herself increasingly at risk for injury by persisting in her decision to walk unassisted. And yet independence is something that Mrs. Rose clearly values a great deal—so it's not clear to me that restraining her against her will *would* actually be in her best interests.

Before giving my own view on the matter, I do think that Mrs. Rose ought to have a thorough physical examination. We certainly want to make sure there isn't some resolvable underlying medical condition precipitating this unsteadiness. Also, it seems to me that, as Mrs. Katz and I were discussing prior to this meeting, Mrs. Rose's situation might benefit from some physical therapy and/or occupational therapy. Alternatively, it may be that as Mrs. Rose suggested a cane, or maybe a walker, might take care of the problem. In short, I think that there are a number of avenues that still warrant exploration.

My own opinion, however, is that even if it turns out to be in Mrs. Rose's best interests to be restrained, as her attending physician I do not feel that it is appropriate for me to sign orders authorizing the use of restraints against her wishes. I think that both the law and the established canon for bioethics is clear: unless there is some reason to think that Mrs. Rose is not competent to make an autonomous decision, the fact that she makes what we think is a bad decision is neither here nor there.

(*As Matthew finishes, Margaret turns to Maureen to give her a look that says, "So there!"*)

BEVERLY: Well, I guess that does it. It seems like the thing to do is for you, Diane, to get together with Margaret and the people in physical and occupational therapy and see what you all can do. Dr. Page, if you're willing, perhaps Maureen can help set up an appointment for her mother. And Margaret, I'll speak with our lawyer and see about getting a form for you to sign that releases County from legal liability should you fall and injure yourself while walking unassisted. It's not the perfect solution, but I guess it'll do until somebody changes the system, eh? But if you have a change of mind, Margaret, we can always make other arrangements.

⑧ A Brief Assessment of the Model

If my arguments have been convincing there is reason to believe not only that autonomous PSR decisions ought to be respected by HCPs but that what generally passes for "respecting autonomy" is but a shadow of what it ought to be. It remains an open question, however, whether one can realistically expect most HCPs to engage patients in the sorts of dialogical interactions outlined in this model.

The progressive change in medicine over the past twenty-five years has led most HCPs to recognize that respecting patients' autonomy should be a major component of responsible health care. But unfortunately few HCPs have any deep understanding of what respecting autonomy means. Nor has there been any concerted attempt to change this situation. It is, of course, notoriously difficulty to teach and evaluate process issues, much less establish their importance for clinical medicine. The science of medicine is considerably more easy to impart than its art. No lab values or specific procedures will ensure that a patient's autonomy is being respected. But as importantly, other sources of resistance impede the project, and what is not clear is how much friction they represent. For example, is the norm for patient-HCP interactions sufficiently flexible to accommodate the deeper, more intimate sorts of interactions that may be called for? Is there ample time for genuine dialogue between patients and HCPs? Are health care institutions, themselves, amenable to the kinds of changes in protocol that might well be necessary? Is there really sufficient concern for respecting patients' autonomy to motivate changes in the way things currently are done?

To a large extent, I think these questions are best answered empirically by creating various clinical models. For whether particular sorts of relationships and interactions between HCPs and patients (that characterize the process of respecting autonomy that has been outlined) are possible will vary with the clinical setting. It may be that a busy urban emergency room will require a very different working model for respecting patients' autonomy than an in-patient ward or a walk-in clinic. A nursing home may need to rethink its staffing or its patient-care protocol in a way that is very different from a hospice or even a different long-term care facility. So no one clinical model will definitively answer the question of whether a dialogical approach to respecting patients' autonomy is realistic. That said, there are reasons to believe that the general model I have laid out is practical.

In the first place, the process I have outlined has as its base the pursuit of better communication and understanding. This means that when done right, engaging in dialogue to respect a patient's autonomy likely *saves* time and therefore money. It does this not just by avoiding errors and promoting a better exchange of information but by assuaging important concerns of patients. For dialogue involves embracing others' concerns as one's own in an attempt to come to terms with their otherness. It is widely recognized that many procedures and diagnostic tests are done (at an enormous cost) in the name of defensive medicine. And yet, what is this fear of litigation rooted in if not failure of the patient-HCP relationship? Obviously, dialogue is not a panacea. Some patients will be argumentative and litigious. But the project of genuinely seeking to understand and address the concerns of patients has as its ordinary consequence the creation of trust, whose balm heals many a wound.

In a related manner, those who can form bonds of trust with their customers gain a competitive market advantage. Satisfaction is a complex concept, but surely it is engendered by a relationship of good faith and confidence, qualities that dialogue and respect for autonomy clearly promote. To the extent that the business of medicine is concerned with the bonds it can form with patients it must be concerned with the dynamics of the relationships that patients experience. Even the poorest of the poor will seek to avoid HCPs who fail to create a relationship of respect.

Perhaps one of the most appealing aspects of the model presented for respecting autonomy is its individual nature and adaptability. An HCP in any environment can engage in the process, irrespective of the professional norm that exists there. This does not mean there are no constraints on what is possible; clearly there are. But even a hectic emergency room or an understaffed nursing home can allow for clinical encounters that promote and respect the exercise of patients' autonomy. Moreover, to the extent that a dialogical approach to respecting patient autonomy gives rise to a healthy, full-bodied patient-HCP relationship, the HCP who is able to establish such relationships will be more effective in many realms of patient care. As has been shown in the corporate environment, an individual's effectiveness ultimately is based in the habits and relationships that she is able to build.[1] How this is related to the superstructure of institutions and particularly managed care is, of course, another matter.

A somewhat different challenge concerns the investment that HCPs are expected to make with each patient. Specifically, is it realistic to expect a nurse or technician or physician or other HCP to develop the interest and invest the energy necessary to genuinely engage each and every patient in dialogue? Part of what distinguishes the various relationships we have are the different levels of intimacy we cultivate and the energy we exert in our encounters with others. So what are we to make of a model that demands such a high level of commitment with each patient? One response simply and unequivocally points to the professional responsibility of HCPs to make a good faith effort to meet patients' medical needs. The professional responsibility of a good teacher is to reach out to each and every child because there is no telling who students will become, no telling which child will be the one who grows up to be president. Similarly, a thorough understanding of patients and their problems is not something to be sought after only for those patients deemed worthy of sufficient effort by particular HCPs. At least in part, professionalism is about treating people fairly and with equal respect, which in the present context demands a good faith effort to form relationships with patients that are meaningful and developed.

A second response to this challenge is that many patient encounters will not require any great investment of energy by HCPs. Patients do not always seek in-depth interactions with HCPs, nor will involved relationships always be necessary for the task at hand. Infirmity can exist on many different levels, some of which may be accessed quite easily. Of course, one must be on one's toes, ready to engage a deeper level if necessary, but it will not always be necessary. Additionally, one's responsibility as an HCP does not require supererogation. Expectations about extending oneself to a patient are limited. Among other things, the professional relationship has parameters. As an HCP one seeks to provide appropriate medical care, part of which involves respecting patients' exercise of autonomy in PSR matters. Self-sacrifice is not a professional responsibility, nor is friendship. And yet the beauty of the dialogical model is that any relationship has the potential to be developed, to become something rich and intensely meaningful. Not a small part of the dissatisfaction with modern medical practice (on both sides of the aisle) revolves around a sense of alienation, with the all too frequent failure to realize relationships that are felt to be genuine and meaningful. So the model presented for respecting autonomy is nonexcessive in its demands of HCPs and it offers the potential to enrich HCPs' experiences with patients.

Dialogue as a means for respecting patient autonomy is practical. As evidenced by the examples in earlier chapters, it is not so distant from normal interaction so as to prove unworkable as a model for clinical interaction. Still, dialogue is truly special, requiring both commitment and attention. Just how one develops the necessary skills to successfully engage in dialogue is, however, another matter.

Drawbacks

Bioethics education—for nurses, physicians, technicians, therapists, and other HCPs—is enormously underdeveloped. Models for education and evaluation within bioethics, though maturing, are notoriously inchoate.[2] Perhaps unavoidably, there is no easy answer for how one goes about educating HCPs about what is involved in respecting patients' autonomy. Clearly, lectures alone will not do, nor will set algorithms, decision trees, or codes of professional conduct. Rather, what is needed is a complex and integrated approach that infuses the concept of respect for autonomy into existing training. It must be incorporated into instruction about taking medical and social histories, conducting physical exams, constructing care plans, and administering treatment. On its most basic level, such an educational approach would remind HCPs (at every step along the way) that the patient as a person must not be forgotten. It would caution HCPs about assuming too much regarding what the patient understands and wishes.

How to realize such a curriculum, however, is not something that as yet I have any answer to. In a recent clinical study conducted with second-year medical students, half of whom received special instruction about the concept of autonomy,[3] no significant differences were observed between the experimental and control groups in terms of their ability to use dialogue to respect patients' autonomous decisions. Presumably, trial and error will help generate and refine an effective educational process for developing HCPs' clinical skills for respecting patients' autonomy. But that my model offers no substantive recommendations is a significant drawback.

An additional drawback touched on earlier has to do with the failure of my model to address the institutional dynamics that so often influence individual behavior. In particular, my discussion has not addressed the patient-care implications of corporate medicine or managed care. It has not discussed the effect of reimbursement schemes that reward an efficiency that is shallow and narrowly conceived. Nor has my discussion examined the fallout (in terms of HCPs' behavior) of strict medical hierarchies that are intolerant of outliers and all who question standard operating procedure.

I did suggest (a la the Covey model) that it is possible for an individual to both transcend accepted paradigms and influence others by modeling behavior that is ultimately more effective in terms of the underlying goals of the activity. But as surely as this is true, it also misses the salient point that outcomes can be overdetermined by existing circumstances. The chances that some HCP can become that one point of light that escapes the gravitational pull of the existing clinical paradigm may be exceedingly small. This may be due to the difficulty in figuring out just how to transcend the existing environment or perhaps the cost of such a project for the individual. But if respecting patients' autonomy is to take root as I have argued it should, institutional and not just individual transformations will be necessary. What forms these institutional changes might take, I have not suggested, nor am I prepared to at this point; and that is a drawback to my model. For institutional policies can undermine individual HCPs' attempts to respect patients' autonomous PSR decisions, and common practices are significantly shaped by environmental forces.

This is not to say, however, that no recourse exists in particular circumstances, save an overhaul of the entire system. One thing that can be done is to put the issues on the table so the barriers can be recognized and discussed, if not dealt with. When financial constraints impede the process of respecting patients' autonomy, say so. When policy decisions make it impossible to realize a full-bodied relationship, call it to the attention of those involved or those in a position to make changes in the system. If a confrontation with a supervisor frustrates appropriate respect for patients' autonomy, acknowledge it. It is not just possible, but genuine, to communicate to a patient (or anyone else) why an appropriate outcome cannot be achieved. Just as dialogue seeks to overcome barriers to understanding by raising them to the level of consciousness and attention, so too is it possible to address systemic or institutional barriers to respecting patients' autonomy.[4] At some level, silence is indeed the voice of complicity.

Afterword: Dialogues Examined

An advantage of presenting dialogues without analysis is that it forces the reader to critique *for herself* the characters and practices described. Moreover, the absence of signposts accurately marking "respect for autonomy" reflects the reality that we observe and participate in every day. It reminds us that individually we must reflect on the interactions we witness and gauge for ourselves the success of this complex project. That said, there is value in considering the criteria employed for our assessments. For it is not altogether obvious how to discern whether an encounter involves a genuine attempt at transformation, a serious search for underlying meaning, and common ground that is developmental and not merely strategic.

To understand where dialogue has succeeded and where it has failed, we must look to see whether an open process of questioning and exploration occurred, whether barriers were acknowledged and attempts made to renegotiate them. Was the interaction educational in its attempt to draw interconnections or was it merely an opportunity to effect a particular outcome? Were individuals prejudged, outcomes predetermined? Was the interaction characterized by a sense of reciprocity and respect and patience? Was there tolerance for alternative viewpoints? Specific to the kinds of encounters portrayed in the preceding dialogues, was there an attempt to orient the patient to the clinical situation and the plans for treatment? Did the various HCPs allow for reinterpretation and renegotiation of their take on the situation? Was feedback solicited? Were there attempts to effect power plays or was there an open and dynamic effort to redefine meaning and projected outcomes? Was there an attempt to come to terms with the "otherness" that (unavoidably) characterizes another person? In proceeding to consider each of the dialogues in turn, the goal is not to measure the performance of any given HCP against some ideal of "respecting autonomy"—for none such exists. Rather, the point is to discern the extent to which various HCPs engaged in a relationship designed to develop a shared understanding of the patient as well as to promote and respect the exercise of that patient's autonomy. The following questions, then, are intended to explore whether in fact such a relationship was entered into and the developmental task undertaken.

Questions

Dialogue 1: An Exception to the Norm

1. In terms of "respecting autonomy," was there something to be gained by pursuing the matter as Brad did, as opposed to simply deferring Tammy's pelvic to an attending physician (preferably a female M.D.)? That is, suppose that as soon as Tammy expressed her resistance Brad simply got a female attending physician to do the pelvic exam. Would that have adequately respected Tammy's autonomous decision?

2. In what ways did Brad help create an interaction that minimized power imbalances? How did Norm Rios's behavior differ in that regard?

3. If we understand their different genders as being a barrier to reaching a shared understanding, to what extent was Brad able to overcome that barrier?

4. Were Brad's open-ended questions sufficient for eliciting Tammy's underlying concerns or should he have gone farther initially?

5. What role does validation of Tammy's feelings and experiences play in Brad's attempt to respect her autonomy?

6. Who defines the central issue of the conflict and how is its definition arrived at?

7. What does Brad state as being of priority and how does that reflect on the matter of respecting Tammy's autonomy?

8. What function is served by Brad's challenging some of Tammy's statements?

9. Assuming that Brad is perfectly competent to perform a professional pelvic exam, does it make a difference whether he is presented as "Brad," "student doctor Aiyam," or "Dr. Aiyam"?

10. In terms of respecting Tammy's autonomy, was there something Joanne could have or should have done?

11. What are some of the institutional impediments to respecting patients' autonomy that present themselves in this setting?

12. As a public aid patient whose care is paid for by society, does Tammy have any special obligations to participate in the public education of physicians in training?

13. Does the fact that Brad and Tammy were strangers create special problems for the project of respecting Tammy's autonomy?

Dialogue 2: A Labor of Love and Respect

1. Given that both Juanita and Jack are intimately involved in this process of childbirth, what weight should Amy give to Jack's values and decisions?

2. Since Juanita had been so adamant in the past about having "natural childbirth," could her actual labor have put her into an altered state of mind that should be overridden?

3. In what sense is Amy renegotiating meaning by referring to "good pain"?

4. In Amy's discussion with Jack, what purpose is served by her validating Juanita's pain?

5. How does the meaning that childbirth has for Jack and Juanita figure into what it means for Amy to respect Juanita's autonomy?

6. What boundaries does Amy set out in terms of managing this childbirth, and how (if at all) does that contribute to the process of respecting autonomy?

7. In virtually any other setting, the kind of pain Juanita is experiencing would be considered entirely unwarranted. Why shouldn't Amy treat Juanita's complaints of pain with the same regard (and swift analgesia) as in other clinical situations?

8. To what extent is it appropriate for Amy to rely so heavily on Juanita's spoken words? Would it be reasonable to judge Juanita's state of mind as well as her preferences by the other cues she provides?

9. How does Amy include Juanita's larger family in the process of respecting Juanita's autonomy?

10. How does Amy construe "interpretation" and "experience" in challenging Juanita's desire for pain medication?

11. Does Amy have a professional responsibility to be something other than neutral in terms of trying to influence Juanita in her decision-making process? And does that conflict with the process of respecting Juanita's autonomy?

12. How does the way that Amy draws out the implications of the various treatment options influence the process of respecting Juanita's autonomy?

13. In terms of respecting Juanita's autonomy, what does it mean for Amy to *encourage* Juanita?

Dialogue 3: Having Final Say

1. How does Stacie elicit Richard's underlying values and concerns?

2. Does Stacie go far enough in exploring Richard's valuation of privacy? In terms of respecting his autonomy, what additional understanding (if any) should she seek regarding Richard's relationship with his wife?

3. Has Richard's thought process (regarding his request of a DNR order) been sufficiently fleshed out by Stacie, or is Kim's interview necessary? If Kim's assessment is important, why wouldn't such psychiatric inquiry be warranted in many more instances of clinical decision-making?

4. Assuming that Richard refused to discuss the matter with Kim, what would be Stacie's obligations in terms of respecting Richard's autonomy?

5. In what ways does Kim challenge Richard's reasoning?

6. What factors in this clinical scenario could be interpreted as realistically undermining Richard's capacity for autonomy?

7. In terms of Stacie's desire to respect Richard's autonomy, how important is it for her to understand the larger context of his decision?

8. In what ways are the power dynamics of the situation Richard finds himself in explored and dealt with?

9. How important is it for Stacie to ensure that Richard understands the implications of his decisions, and does she do an adequate job of it?

10. What are Kim's and Stacie's intentions, and are they made plain?

11. Can Stacie genuinely respect Richard's autonomy without getting input from the community that has helped define who he is—particularly his wife, Betty?

12. To what extent is the PSR nature of Richard's request discussed and resolved?

13. Given Sara's apprehensions about the autonomous nature of Richard's decision (along with the lack of opportunity for her to explore the matter, given the emergency situation she found herself in), was she right to simply have acceded to the existing DNR order? After all, a man's life was at stake.

Dialogue 4: Protecting Respect

1. In what ways do Robert and Albert recognize that a person's capacity for autonomy can be vulnerable? Are there significant differences between their respective appreciations for this vulnerability, and how do their differences play out clinically?

2. Why does Robert wish to diminish the import attributed to Herman's previous behavior, and is Robert justified in doing so?

3. How does reliance on verbal responses, as opposed to other cues, influence what it means to respect Herman's autonomy? Is there something amiss in Robert's reliance on this singular representation of Herman's beliefs, values, concerns, and desires?

4. When Albert admonishes his son to *really listen* in his dealings with Linda and Herman, what is Albert referring to, and what does it mean to *really listen?*

5. What is gained in terms of autonomy by pushing Herman as Robert wishes to?

6. How do the patient's own expectations contribute to what it means to respect autonomy? What difference does it make if such expectations run counter to what is accepted practice for confidentiality, truth-telling, and so forth?

7. Given the dynamics in the case, what does it mean to regard Herman's health care decisions as PSR? Moreover, who should play a role in defining how PSR gets interpreted?

8. At what points does the dialogue with Herman take a developmental emphasis as opposed to a (merely) strategic emphasis?

9. Clearly, much of what is at issue in this case is protecting, promoting, and respecting Herman's autonomy. Also at issue, however, is Linda's desire to work within well-established parameters that constitute a "comfort zone" for everyone involved. What (if any) regard should Robert have for this desire to stay within the comfort zone?

10. Does Robert adequately appreciate and deal with the role that fear plays in Herman's existence?

11. What underlying issues does Robert bring out into the open for discussion?

12. Robert in essence has argued that it is inappropriate to prejudge the developmental potential for any given dialogue—in this case, the extent to which the interaction might help Herman deal with and hopefully overcome his fears. But given the risks associated with the present gambit, is Robert justified in pushing the issue?

13. Is it really the case, as Albert suggests at the end of the dialogue, that Herman's response will determine whether Robert and Albert did the right thing?

Dialogue 5: Restraint by Any Other Name

1. To what extent do the multitude of institutional barriers to providing a safe and independent environment excuse health care providers for the restrictions they impose on nursing home residents?

2. What are the institutional barriers to fostering genuine dialogue regarding the concerns of nursing home residents?

3. Do the nursing home staff members regard their residents as deserving a different status than themselves in terms of independence, input in

decision-making, and so forth? In what sense is that different status justified?

4. Margaret accuses her daughter of not understanding. Who (if anyone) truly does understand the situation that Margaret finds herself in?

5. How is the decision regarding the initial PRN restraint order handled, and what (if anything) is problematic about it?

6. Does the fact that Margaret entered County *voluntarily* play any role in terms of how County's policies regarding restraints should or should not apply to her?

7. Who asks Margaret *real* questions, as opposed to makes statements or gives orders merely phrased in the form of questions?

8. To what extent does the relative lack of imagination exhibited with regard to problem-solving in this scenario constitute a failure of respecting autonomy?

9. Did not allowing Margaret to participate in the entire meeting constitute a failure in respecting her autonomy?

10. In what ways were Margaret's views, values, and concerns acknowledged and seriously considered? How were they invalidated or minimized?

11. How was the matter of power introduced and handled? What attempts were made to negotiate a balance in the power dynamics?

12. In terms of Margaret's autonomy, what is the importance of her being reasonable? That is, what is the relation between Margaret being judged reasonable and what is involved in respecting her autonomy?

13. In terms of how the various HCPs interact with Margaret, what distinguishes how Matthew engages her?

Notes

Chapter 1: The Setup

1. Clearly, this is not an exhaustive, totalizing, or exclusive conception of education. Many alternatives stress other aspects of education, from perceptual to behavioral. This said, the notion that education involves the development of a deeper sense of understanding seems in many ways a core meaning of education. To defend this claim, however, would take me beyond the scope of the present work.

2. Susan Wolf (1992:32).

3. Throughout this book *our* will refer to Western society. Outside of Western culture, where notions such as identity and responsibility are more closely connected with the concept of community, I am less certain about the importance of autonomy.

4. See Gaylin and Jennings (1996). The kindest interpretation I can give of this work is that its authors mean to denounce a variety of common misinterpretations regarding the meaning of autonomy, as well as the proper place and value of its exercise. That said, the more obvious reading is that "autonomy" represents anything willed by a human being, that "respect for autonomy" entails kow-towing to such expressions of will, and that as a consequence of this understanding we should deemphasize the value our society places on autonomy.

5. See Levi (1996).

6. The notion that the physician represents the "paradigm health care provider" is both widely assumed and deeply problematic. Still, because physicians' behavior often sets the tone for the practice of medicine, I think it is useful to call attention to the noneducational aspects of their training in particular. For a recent litany of such shortcomings, see Stewart Wolf (1997).

7. Of course, medicine is not alone in its tendency to zealously embrace hierarchical tradition, but it does so with a pretension of objectivity that in the face of medicine's ideological stance and position in society certainly deserves to be more severely challenged.

8. As anyone familiar with domination knows, this may take more or less subtle forms. Social de facto domination is just as real as domination resulting from de jure exclusion or discrimination.

9. Crapanzano (1990:276).

10. Burbules (1993:xii).

11. Burbules has developed a general account of such relationships, and the char-

acterization that I provide here is based largely on this account. This said, my concern with dialogue is significantly different from Burbules's. Drawing from the work of Freire, Gadamer, and Habermas, Burbules provides an extensive analysis and characterization of the rules that regulate dialogue, the values and attitudes that make dialogue successful, and the distinct genres that dialogue can manifest. His concern is to show dialogue's potential for transcending the divisions that exist in a pluralistic society as well as the power imbalances that plague society. Moreover, Burbules argues that it is "the fabric of dialogical interchange that sustains the very capacity to generate and revise" the answers, solutions, and agreements found in human history (1993:144). Additionally Burbules claims that because such outcomes are always provisional, it is all the more important to sustain the (dialogical) process by which they are reached and revised. Thus, Burbules's project is both complex and expansive. In drawing from this rather involved and sophisticated account, I want to make clear that my concern with dialogue is much more limited. I merely want to explain the role that dialogue can play in clinical situations that concern personal autonomy. In subsequent chapters I will flesh out how dialogue can function as a means for discerning the existence of autonomy, for promoting the exercise of personal autonomy, and as an intervention in cases of conflict. What follows here, though, is a brief discussion of how dialogue, as a general concept, is distinct from other types of discourse and what its particular characteristics connote.

12. Burbules (1993:42).

13. It strikes me that the distinction between being committed to one's fellow participants and having concern for them is an important one, especially for HCPs who might be skeptical of embracing dialogue as a model for respecting patients' exercise of autonomy. The distinction I have in mind is this: *Being committed to* another involves actually caring for her and being interested in continuing one's relationship with her. By contrast, *having concern for* another may involve no more than being concerned to understand her—where this may serve primarily strategic purposes.

14. This recommendation has been advanced by Quill and Brody (1996).

15. Because I find it useful to have someone in mind when I think of "an individual in the abstract," I will refer periodically to Sally. Sally is about forty years old, slender, five foot five, with shoulder-length blond hair. Sally has a wonderfully friendly smile and a South Carolina accent and walks her dogs in my neighborhood. I think it is important to remember that there is no such thing as "the individual" sans particular qualities, attributes, characteristics. By referring to Sally, I continually remind myself that "the individual" is always someone real, with feelings, concerns, and a unique personality.

16. Articulated by David DeGrazia (1992), specified principlism is an approach in which one begins with general principles and then modifies them as needed (by casuistic methodology), using something like wide reflective equilibrium (cf. Rawls 1971) to justify proposed modifications.

Chapter 2: Background

1. Gaylin (1996:45).
2. Clement (1996:16).
3. This is an amended version of Paul Hershey's (1985:71) characterization that posits the following two conditions as necessary and sufficient to define a paternalistic act: the paternalistic action is primarily intended to benefit the recipient and the recipient's consent or dissent is not a relevant consideration for the initiator. It seems to me that the emendation is necessary, for according to Hershey's characterization if one gives any consideration whatsoever to the recipient's wishes one is no longer acting paternalistically, and this seems wrong. Surely paternalism is not negated merely by an agent recognizing the wishes of the recipient. The recipient's consent or dissent need not be, as Hershey claims, entirely irrelevant to one's motivation for acting. In the context of Hershey's definition, all that is required to ensure paternalism is that the recipient's wishes not be of primary or overriding concern.
4. For example, a four-year-old child's wishes about taking penicillin for her pneumonia do not deserve equal consideration. Similarly, most would agree that if the intended beneficiary is clearly irrational, her wishes do not deserve equal respect either—though this is not to say that they deserve no respect at all.
5. Trilling (1950:221).
6. Bronchoscopy involves inserting a catheter (about the diameter of a Tootsie Roll) down the patient's throat and into the air passages of the respiratory system to visualize and often biopsy those air passages. A lumbar puncture involves inserting a large bore needle (about the size of a large pencil lead) through the skin of the lower back into the spinal column to sample spinal fluid for pathogens and unusual fluid composition. A myelogram involves inserting contrast medium into the spinal fluid and then doing radiological studies to visualize the integrity of the spinal canal, nerve roots, and bony or cartilaginous structures.
7. Only the strictest utilitarian would argue that *all* our decisions are open to such challenge. Whether Sally should get chocolate sprinkles on her ice cream is not of sufficient consequence for most of us to warrant our concern, much less our intervention.
8. At various points in history the will has been identified with appetites (Hobbes), with reason (Kant), and as an intermediary between the two (Plato, Aristotle, Aquinas).
9. See Peters (1967:30–46).
10. It might appear to beg the question to attribute this interpretation to Hobbes, given his deterministic approach. Hobbes understood, however, that individuals can behave voluntarily, for otherwise he could not have appealed to the importance of obligation and contract in his psychological and political doctrines.
11. "So for Spinoza, as indeed for Freud, rational self-understanding is the key to self-determination—to ego-autonomy" (Benn 1988:189).

12. Mill did not believe that living autonomously was *logically* necessary to max-imize happiness, but rather that it was necessary in a practical sense. Specifically, Mill argued that living autonomously conduces to an individual's growth and de-velopment and that, generally, it is the most reliable mechanism for identifying and satisfying one's best interests.

13. Hill (1987:133).

14. Feinberg (1986:chap. 18).

15. An objection to invoking ideal autonomy at all is the Deweyan cry that it perpetuates the quest for certainty and thereby reinforces the counterproductive belief that *real* self-government exists only under certain rather isolated conditions. While I have some sympathy for this point of view I think that, postmodernism aside, we *do* work on the assumption that most people are autonomous. So while the concept of ideal autonomy does transcend the normal condition (what Stan-ley Benn has called autarchy), the value and importance we attribute to being au-tonomous devolves on the normal condition, not the ideal condition. I recognize that in some sense this response begs the question whether the normal condition of autonomy is the basis for various important values. My hope is that the remain-der of my arguments will be convincing on this issue.

16. For a thorough account of the concept of freedom see Benn (1988, esp. chap. 7).

17. Morton White (1973) explains that free action can be formulated logically as follows, where *P* stands for some predicate and represents the normative aspect of freedom:

Sally did A freely   is equivalent to   *~Necessary (Sally was P → Sally did A)*

This means that if Sally was P, in a given social or historical context, being P would not count as a "good excuse" for doing A; i.e., it would not absolve Sally of respon-sibility.

18. For the original articulation of freedom as a three-place relation see MacCal-lum (1967).

19. Contrast this with "Your money or I'll spit on your shoe." Obviously this normative aspect of freedom will give rise to disputes over *when* a person is free to choose. In part the nature of such disputes is captured in Isaiah Berlin's (1969) dis-tinction between positive and negative freedom as well as in debates over what constitutes a reasonable "price to pay" for a given choice. A more full-bodied and quite interesting exegesis of freedom, discussed specifically in relation to autono-my, is carried out by Berofsky (1995:34–76). He provides a summary of four dis-tinct senses of freedom, where what he calls *volitional freedom* captures the nor-mative component I am referring to here (52).

20. Imagine, for example, that Sally is held down and tickled until she pees on herself. In this instance a generally autonomous action, urination, is made nonau-tonomous due to a state of unfreedom. One can also imagine Sally having been

shackled to a wall in the hot sun for days to the point that she becomes truly delusional and thereby loses the mental functioning that makes her autonomous.

Chapter 3: Characterizing Autonomy

1. That is, "with the right kind of cause." See Parfit (1986:271). The distinction between psychological connectedness and physical identity can be illustrated as follows. Imagine that Sally, while out walking her dogs, has a transformational experience that involves a complete break with her former self. Though she remains five foot five, slender, with shoulder-length blond hair, and in possession of two moderately well-behaved canines, she now has an entirely different set of memories, interests, and values compared with those possessed by the person who only minutes earlier was known as Sally. Parfit's point amounts to the claim that because what matters (from a metaphysical and a moral standpoint) is the degree of psychological connectedness, *Sally* no longer exists. That is to say, because there remains nothing beyond the physical identity to link Sally with this new being, we should regard this new being as a separate and distinct person. Parfit's arguments are both enormously rich and complex, but for the present discussion, the salient point is that it is psychological connectedness and continuity that confers on individuals the opportunity to be regarded as morally distinguishable, and to exist over time.

2. For Parfit this means that "a person's existence just consists in the existence of a brain and a body, and the occurrence of a series of interrelated physical and mental events" (1986:211).

3. Feinberg (1986:28).

4. That is, if it is necessary to be consistent, logical, and truthful to qualify as rational, then all sorts of human behavior would fail to qualify as rational and hence could not be considered autonomous. Given the general character of human behavior, such a requirement threatens to relegate autonomy to a very limited realm in our lives. For a discussion of this issue, see Susan Wolf (1992).

5. See Benn's requirements for autarchy (1976:116).

6. An example of this is Benn's argument that an aspect of practical rationality is that beliefs and their related inferences may entail certain action commitments. "Believing today is Wednesday does seem to commit us not to say 'Today is Tuesday.' Now as one proceeds from the epistemic commitment to moral, political, and religious ones, the implications become less tight; that is, they are more open to doubt and disagreement. Still, the language of implication is not out of order" (1988:30–31).

7. For example, imagine a search committee member, Jake, who continually uses the pronoun *he* to refer to the next program director, despite the fact that no one has been chosen. When another search committee member points out this usage there may well be disagreements about how Jake's behavior should be interpreted, what it should count as evidence for, and what inferences may be drawn from it. But this does not mean that people disagree about what the evidence *is* or what

legitimates an inference. It merely means that there are different beliefs about what Jake's behavior stands for, differences that, presumably, could be cleared up given sufficient time and adequate communication. That there are different interpretations of Jake's behavior does not mean that some people are not comprehending the situation.

8. Where to set this minimum threshold is itself a matter of great concern. See Wikler (1979).

9. For a related discussion that reaches a different sort of conclusion, see Betty Cox White (1994). In her analysis of the concept of competence, White argues that whenever competence is being considered the analysis should be framed in terms of specific competences, as opposed to general competence. White also holds that competence should be understood as a matter of degree, not a threshold determination. To the extent that White's analysis is limited to an assessment of an individual's ability to perform a given task, I think her conclusions are not problematic. The extension of her analysis into the moral realm, however, is far from straightforward. In the first place, the sum of individual competences may be considerably larger than their individual parts, hence warranting a general designation of competence. In the second place, it is not clear that beyond a given threshold it makes sense to speak of greater degrees of competency generating a higher (or even different) moral standing. That White believes there is an affective component to competence only compounds the problematic nature of extending her analysis into the moral realm. For then one faces the troubling implication that there is a median level of affect, above and below which one's moral standing is lessened in proportion to one's deviation from "the proper amount."

10. See Feinberg (1986:156–58) for an interesting and sensitive discussion of coercive pressure.

11. In fact, describing autonomy in terms of a decision-making process is itself misleading insofar as it implies that autonomy always involves active, conscious, directed decision-making. Nonetheless, given that autonomy is grounded in the ability to carry out a critical evaluation and be able to revise one's ends or goals on the basis of that evaluation, the language of decision-making is perhaps the most appropriate.

12. Bernard Gert and Timothy Duggan (1979:203) formulate this requirement as follows: One must "have the ability to believe that there are coercive and non-coercive incentives both for doing X and for not doing X" and tend to act in accordance with one's beliefs about these incentives.

13. Though often such issues are phrased in terms of *competency,* the ambiguity of this term makes it problematic. For some (e.g., Beauchamp 1991) competency refers simply to the ability to perform a given task, for others (e.g., Erde 1991; Knight 1991; Schaffner 1991) it denotes a general level of functioning that society judges acceptable. For still others (e.g., Morreim 1991; Pincoffs 1991; Wikler 1979) it is a global determination equivalent to *being autonomous.* Betty Cox White (1994) has gone some distance in clarifying the concept of competence, but the transferabili-

ty of her analysis into the moral (as opposed to the merely descriptive) realm is highly problematic. The discussion that follows in part responds to her position.

14. I have in mind debilities such as memory problems, losses of association (where certain cause-and-effect relations are no longer realized), inability to control particular impulses, impaired sense of time, and so forth.

15. Clearly, the physical analogy should be taken only so far, since purely physical capacities play no morally significant role in the origination or maintenance of the capacity for autonomy, and so their absence alone will not diminish it. Certain physical incapacities, such as blindness or deafness, may impair comprehension by limiting an individual's perceptions, but if a person is informed, or deliberately chooses to remain uninformed, such incapacities do not by themselves impair the capacity for autonomy.

16. Presumably, one could map out areas of critical evaluation and decision-making that would be affected by specific incapacities, and depending on their nature and extent redraw the appropriate bounds of autonomous behavior. Obviously, this can get very complicated if one is not careful to separate out the "capacity to govern oneself" from the "actual condition of autonomy" from the "right to govern oneself." Imagine Sally is an autonomous person who once she starts eating pasta becomes psychologically unable to control how much she eats. In mapping out the bounds of autonomous behavior, pasta eating would not be included as part of the *actual condition* of autonomy, for literally Sally is unable to control herself once she has begun. But Sally is generally autonomous, that is, able to formulate, revise, and pursue her ends or goals. Thus, so long as Sally is aware that she will experience an overwhelming desire once she has begun to eat pasta, Sally has the capacity to make an autonomous decision whether to begin to eat pasta. Thus, pasta eating *would be* included when mapping the *capacity* to govern herself. A further complication would be if *prior* to Sally's decision she experienced a very strong desire to eat pasta. Here, to map autonomous behavior we would need to examine more closely the process of her decision-making. It is in part due to such practical difficulties that I reject the process of decision-making as the locus of concern for autonomy.

17. For an interesting discussion of fear-induced akrasia, see McKnight (1993).

18. For a critique of psychiatry as legitimating such a political witch-hunt, see Szasz (1970). Clearly, the use of a threshold does not avoid this problem entirely. Still, the demand for a single defensible standard does mitigate against the worst abuses by at least proscribing capriciousness.

19. For example, linguists have long argued that learning a language, any language, is one of the most complex cognitive tasks humans ever encounter. If this is the case, then it says a great deal about people's native potential for intellectual development.

20. See Elster (1982). For those unfamiliar with this old fable, the fox sees a bunch of grapes that he wants, but try as he might, he just cannot reach them. Angry at his failure, he walks away grumbling that they were probably sour anyway.

21. Clearly, this pertains to our individual aspirations, but by logical extension it also should hold for our (more abstract) ideas about justice, equality, rationality, and so on.

22. As my good friend Howard Aizenstein has reminded me, *the point* of deliberation could be simply the enjoyment one gets from the activity. This said, what could deliberation contribute *beyond* enjoyment?

23. Clearly, how we should understand children in this regard is extremely problematic, for the capacities that make autonomy possible develop over time and may be more or less present in any given child.

24. For an argument that even utilitarianism depends on the autonomous nature of decisions and actions if they are to have value, see Haworth (1986:136–47).

Chapter 4: Kinds of Autonomy

1. People can and regularly do behave in ways that are inconsistent with their true beliefs, their genuine values, and their intentions, whether due to compulsion, weakness of will, basic error, or something else.

2. Richards (1981:11).

3. Haworth (1986:22–46).

4. For a superb survey article laying out current discussions about autonomy, see Christman (1988).

5. Christman (1988:112).

6. Christman (1987).

7. See Berofsky (1995:99–103).

8. "When certain desires explain the dictates of reason and occupy a central place in the economy of a person's life, why choose the desires *endorsed* by reason rather than those which explain the endorsement, when they are in conflict?" (Berofsky 1995:101).

9. "The insistence that the self is to be identified with the rational, epistemically inaccessible, conscious system makes sense when that system is also assumed to play the crucial role in explaining our behavior and our experience. But when that assumption is abandoned, it seems plausible to shift to the idea that the self incorporates whatever elements play a central role in the true explanatory theory of behavior and experience" (Berofsky 1995:103).

10. Gerald Dworkin (1988:15). Feinberg (1986:113–27) employs a similar move by characterizing particular decisions in terms of their voluntariness and setting out conditions that impugn not autonomy, per se, but the possibility of voluntariness.

11. For his part Dworkin does not endorse this inference. But unless we are to revisit the problem of incompleteness, discussed above, it is not clear how else we can question the autonomy of Sally's decisions other than by asking whether somehow her capacity to be autonomous has been compromised.

12. In the Dworkin/Frankfurt model, this would entail creating HODs that identify with LODs.

13. "We must remind ourselves that even an honest judgment can be a relative-

ly shallow one, that although one can realize that it would be a good thing not to act on a desire, the significance of the desire can far surpass that of the reasoned judgment, and only the philosopher's traditional preference for the rational or the cognitive blurs philosophical vision and generates a misleading conception of the self" (Berofsky 1995:104). "Unless we suppose that we are always what we would like to be—a foolish assumption—we have to concede that a person may have to acknowledge as his own a desire he would prefer to be rid of or disclaim a desire he actually has, no matter how intimate the desire presents itself as. . . . A doctrine which fails to acknowledge a potential gap between the actual self and the ego ideal is incapable of comprehending the tragedy of a life judged a failure by the one who lived it" (Berofsky 1995:220).

14. Gerald Dworkin (1988:16) puts this nicely when he describes autonomy as "a feature that evaluates a whole way of living one's life [that] can only be assessed over extended portions of a person's life." This again points out the inadequacy of Betty Cox White's (1994) reliance on specific determinations of competence to ground our moral conception of autonomy.

15. For an interesting discussion of this issue with regard to cults, see Davis (1986:131–93).

16. An example might be a person absent-mindedly eating tortilla chips while engaged in a conversation.

17. See Gerald Dworkin (1988:17).

18. Ellul (1973:vi).

19. Nor is this problem overcome by abandoning the "true self" as the locus of autonomy and instead identifying *objective evaluation* as the determinant for whether autonomy is extant—as suggested by Berofsky (1995). For the question remains how either to conceptualize such independence/objectivity or to gauge its authenticity, that is, its genuine objectivity.

Parenthetically, moving the "true" nature of autonomy to some idealized condition of "objective evaluation" introduces some potentially troubling and serious issues. Specifically, Who defines what counts as an ideally constituted and executed evaluation? What counts as a sufficiently objective evaluation such that it warrants our respect? How will particular evaluations (in the real world—say, patient care settings) be judged, and by whom—which clearly admits of infinite regress? If we are to take seriously Berofsky's model these concerns are not trivial.

20. We know from experience that sometimes things need to be brought to our attention many times before we consciously appreciate their relevance and begin to seriously address them. What *brings* them to our consciousness? It is very unclear.

21. See Dewey (1957:163–77; 1987:243–87).

22. See, for example, Moody (1989).

23. For an early article in this vein, see Taylor (1979).

24. With regard to autonomy, this would mean that because the right to be self-governing depends upon the capacity to be self-governing, which in turn depends

upon a variety of complex social relations that necessarily involve belonging and obligation, it is inconsistent to respect the right to be self-governing without also protecting (and, in fact, promoting) the conditions and relations that give rise to the capacity. Adding support to this view is Ian Shapiro's historical critique of liberal rights theory (1988). In his work Shapiro argues that the idea of libertarian independence is founded on the economic myth that if left to itself the competitive market is the perfect mechanism for promoting individual and social development. By exposing this "natural" model as a myth, Shapiro challenges the basis for supporting (or aspiring to) an individualistic conception of society. A different approach for justifying the commitment to care for others is advanced by Robert Goodin (1985) and discussed in the context of autonomy by Grace Clement (1996:73–75).

25. Benhabib (1987:158).

26. See Bernstein (1991:231).

27. By "principled" I do not mean to imply that being autonomous entails having good or virtuous principles, much less acting on them. Sally is certainly no less autonomous for being evil or leading a wicked life. I mean only that being autonomous entails living one's life according to some principles that one has the capacity to examine and revise. Similarly, by "responsible" I mean only that Sally has the properties that make her responsible for her actions.

28. See Habermas (1984) for a discussion of the conditions necessary for legitimately achieving consensus.

29. Obviously, attempts to avoid compartmentalizing or isolating particular concerns can go a long way toward resolving disputes. It is also clear that certain attitudes, like "It's *my* decision and no one else's business!" often make otherwise manageable disputes unresolvable. But some disputes are genuinely intractable—often over values—and in these cases decision-making must collapse into one of two alternatives: either it belongs to the individual or it belongs to someone else.

30. It is outside the scope of my project to discuss how various relationships situate autonomy such that it can play its foundational role for concepts such as moral equality, respect, justice, and so forth.

31. Benn (1988:119–20). For a general discussion of this issue, see 112–21.

Chapter 5: The Future of Autonomy

1. For if actions *cannot* be both imprudent and autonomous, this question regarding present versus future autonomy becomes either a straightforward paternalistic question of whether we should override someone's nonautonomous preferences to secure her future autonomy or a question about what grounds justify paternalistically overriding someone's autonomous preferences, given that the grounds can no longer be that the action is imprudent. In other words, in the absence of imprudence is some criterion sufficient to warrant overriding someone's autonomous preferences?

2. Most notably, various religions proscribe self-debasing or self-injurious activities on the grounds that one has a responsibility to the self one will become.

3. See Parfit (1986, esp. part 3).

4. Lawrence Haworth's rejoinder (1986:136–47) that the well-being utilitarians seek to maximize must be *autonomous* well-being does assuage this objection, but in the process defeats the current argument that well-being should trump the exercise of autonomy.

5. Dewey (1957:244–54). We do need to be clear that we are talking about individuals who are autonomous, for there may be special considerations when dealing with either those who have yet to (fully) develop autonomy (e.g., children) or who drift in an out of autonomous states.

6. Related to this, of course, is Mill's argument that to sustain the capacity for autonomy it is necessary to be allowed to live an autonomous life, that is, to have one's autonomous PSR decisions respected.

7. A different approach for defending this general claim that respect for a person (in certain cases) may entail overriding present autonomous decisions involves replacing *autonomy* with *authenticity* as the object of our concern (see Welie 1994). What is not at all clear, however, is why concern for consistency, previous patterns of behavior, or even a well-established value system should de jure override an (admittedly) autonomous decision that breaks with tradition. Granted, radical breaks constitute red flags warranting further investigation, but the present is where we do our living, not the past.

8. For example, if Frances and Floyd unknowingly ingest a poison and Floyd purges the toxin by vomiting, from one perspective we can say that Floyd is worse off than Frances, but from a different perspective that Floyd is better off than Frances. What makes this contradiction apparent is that we are conflating two different frames of reference. Another example, one that does not use the concept of well-being, is this: when we gauge a person's degree of understanding by her lack of confusion, it is only an *apparent* contradiction that third-year graduate students seem more confused than first-year undergraduates about the meaning of a right. There is no *real* contradiction because we are no longer using the same frame of reference for *confusion,* and hence *understanding.* The issue for the undergraduate is What is a right?; the issue for the graduate student is What does it mean to speak in terms of rights?

9. Such a scheme would be like promoting fertility on the grounds that maximizing the number of children is valuable regardless of how they are raised or lead their lives.

10. It is a separate question whether respecting autonomy commits one to *promoting* autonomy.

11. Parfit (1986:319).

12. It seems to me that if it is wrong to commit others to irrevocable conditions, then it is only incidental to Parfit's argument whether those conditions are good

or bad—though obviously it will matter to the concerned parties. Since part of what Parfit wants to do is break down the self-other dichotomy, it may be mistaken to even rely on the notion of "what it is *wrong* to do to others."

13. Parfit (1986:321).

14. For a general discussion of our obligations to protect the future interests of children, see Feinberg (1980).

Chapter 6: Appreciating Autonomy

1. Though not the first to have expressed this critique, Thomas Kuhn stands out as having formalized the claim that "there is no neutral algorithm for theory choice, no systematic decision procedure which, properly applied, must lead each individual in the group to the same decision" (1970:200). For a discussion of Kuhn's argument that the development of disciplines (rightly) considered rational has depended on behavior previously thought irrational, see Bernstein (1991:59).

2. Imagine, for example, a shy and submissive Sally who suddenly risks her own physical well-being to protect her children, be it from her abusive husband or a violent criminal who has intruded on their lives.

3. See Parfit (1986:313).

4. At least for those of us in Western society.

5. Sally has integrity insofar as she is faithful to her own moral convictions and principles, where *her own* means that her moral convictions and principles are "rooted in [her] own character, and not merely inherited" (Feinberg 1986:36). Integrity thus presupposes moral authenticity, not in the sense of inventing the moral law for oneself, but in the sense of endorsing (one's) moral law. Such an endorsement involves reflecting, balancing, and compromising among the competing concerns that inevitably arise in connection with moral laws. Thus conceived, integrity clearly supposes that Sally is autonomous. For only as an autonomous person can Sally critically reexamine, balance, and be faithful to the moral convictions and principles she has embraced.

6. For a discussion of autonomy's primacy for ascriptions of praise, blame, responsibility, dignity and self-esteem, see Haworth (1986:136–47).

7. Robert White (1959) discusses possible explanations for autonomy's basic value, including its capacity for promoting species survival (315), its representing "an inborn drive to do and learn how to do" (307), and its reflecting a innate desire to stand out as an individual (324).

8. The suggestion is Wright Neely's; the quotation is from Haworth (1986:188).

9. Obviously this does not mean that overriding Sally's autonomous decisions is incompatible with *valuing* her autonomy, given that harm to others can be a perfectly good reason for overriding autonomous decisions.

10. Dewey (1957:252).

11. Mill (1947:chap. 3, par. 3; see also chap. 1, par. 11.)

12. It is important to bear in mind that the paternalist position being discussed here cannot sidestep the issue by saying, "Most of the time exercising autonomy

has value in terms of well-being, but not this time." For unless paternalists can present a universally agreed-upon schema for when exercising autonomy is and is not valuable (and none such exists), I have already argued that the value of exercising autonomy must reside in the present. Thus valuing the present exercise of autonomy is an all-or-nothing concept.

13. Though the social policy implications are far more complex, a similar argument might be made with the decision of a pregnant woman to drink alcohol.

14. Donald VanDeVeer (1986:69) points out that since subsequent consent is not regarded as justification in cases of *non*-paternalistic intervention, it is not at all clear why paternalists should hold special status. To illustrate his point, VanDeVeer constructs the following two cases. "First, suppose that you are knocked unconscious by a gang of hoodlums; at a later time you realize that had it not occurred you would have boarded a plane as you had intended, one which exploded and left no survivors. In retrospect you 'are glad' that you were knocked out. Consider a second case. Suppose that you are a woman who was raped when she was eighteen. The experience was devastating and the next few years an enormous struggle, psychologically and otherwise. Seventeen years later, at thirty-five, you judge that, in some sense, it was 'good' that the rape occurred. This last remark strikes one as incredible. What could be meant? Suppose that, in spite of a difficult life, there is something that has made your life one of deep happiness for over a decade, namely, the loving and joyous relationship which you have experienced with the two daughters born of the trauma at eighteen. You might be able to say that your life is much happier than it would have been if numerous other sequences had occurred; in that sense and in that sense only you have a positive attitude toward the set of prior events. But none of this supports the view that the rape was consented to, permissible, or not a heinous wrong."

15. Some written accounts of Cowart's experiences have been collected in Kliever (1991). In addition, two very powerful short documentary films about the case can be obtained from the organization Concern for Dying, based in New York City. *Please Let Me Die* chronicles Cowart's case during his hospitalization in 1974, while *Dax's Case* takes up his story ten years later and includes interviews with Cowart, his mother, and various physicians and lawyers involved in his case. For discussions about autonomy, these two films serve as provocative tools, especially if group discussion takes place *before* Cowart's outcome is made clear in the second film.

16. For a discussion of this see Childress (1983:chap. 3).

17. Scoccia (1990).

18. One thing this points to is the inadequacy of the term *primarily self-regarding,* since it is natural to assume that something cannot be primarily self-regarding if it significantly affects others.

19. See Ronald Dworkin (1978:198).

20. Similar logic is used by some critics of capital punishment—that the state should not have the power to perform certain actions, even when they might be warranted.

21. Specifically, the concern is with who gets to decide which, and whose, PSR autonomous decisions get overridden. What if I autonomously decide to float from desire to desire, to experience life in its most immediate, sensual, and unreflective forms? Are my desires any less valuable? My autonomous decision any less deserving of respect? If I have the capacity to choose, why should I not be allowed to abdicate my decision-making? Who are you, or anyone else for that matter, to tell me how reflective I must be? These seem to me to be reasonable responses. And yet my guess is that should an intellectual, expert-oriented elite possess the power to decide which PSR decisions get overridden, responses such as these will be rejected.

22. By "unencumbered" I do not mean that other individuals or society at large should not try to influence the person at all, only that whatever influence is exerted must acknowledge and respect the wishes of the autonomous person who is making the PSR decision.

23. One attempt to address this issue is Betty Cox White's formulation of "affective competence," whereby individuals are considered *competent* (ostensibly, a prerequisite for being autonomous) if and only if they are able to perceive and attend to their emotions in an appropriate manner. Presumably, this could be amended to account for a maturational component of autonomy, but such a stipulation appears to remain essentially ad hoc. See White (1994, esp. chap. 4).

24. Gerald Dworkin (1988:7).

25. Siegler (1985).

26. An example of an article that is at once quite reasoned and quite blind to the major issue of autonomy is David Thomasma's sensitive discussion of how attitudes of beneficence as well as other psychological factors make doctor-patient relationships more than just legal, economic, and contractual arrangements. In particular Thomasma claims that because people who are sick need help, "their rights to autonomy should not get in the way of their physical needs" (1983:243). Is Thomasma suggesting that rights involving autonomy or justice or equality or fairness are things to be disregarded for a "better outcome?" The tendency to introduce ad hoc premises like "promoting health is more important than respecting autonomy" undercut the validity, if not the soundness, of such arguments.

Chapter 7: The Landscape of Autonomy

1. As Margaret Battin (1991) points out, for many people the notion of a "natural death" is laden with Hollywood stereotypes often not borne out by reality. It takes but a few encounters with dying people to realize that "natural death" may be very far indeed from the "painless, conscious, dignified, culminative slipping-away" that many people imagine it to be.

2. Because simply seeking information appears to be neutral with regard to respecting autonomous decisions, it is not even clear whether (on PSR grounds) Leo can prohibit informational question asking—though, of course, he may choose (on PSR grounds) to not respond to questions.

By speaking of "informational question asking," I mean to distinguish questions intended to gather information from questions intended to, say, give unwanted advice, be manipulative, or effect some other end that the person (whose autonomous PSR decision is at issue) is known to be opposed to. So, for example, were Shaun to ask a question of Leo's daughter that effectively breached confidentiality regarding Leo's prostate condition, it might be proscribed on PSR grounds.

3. Note that the nature of HCPs' role makes their professional responsibility specific to matters of health. Thus, Shaun has a professional responsibility to promote only Leo's health status, not his financial status or his love life or anything else. Still, the boundaries of *health* are sufficiently fuzzy to allow for a variety of interpretations for what counts as within the realm of promoting it.

4. Though dialogues, like all encounters, have at least two sides, currently I am not concerned with patients' responsibilities to the clinical relationship. Clearly, patients must be more than passive recipients if they mean to promote their health. They must communicate clearly and work to focus their energies in productive ways. But it is not at all clear that patients have, as some claim, definite responsibilities to promote their own health. Such misgivings regarding patients' actual responsibilities combined with the importance of respecting autonomy and the fact that HCPs generally hold much greater power in clinical encounters have led me to focus on the norms and behavior of HCPs rather than patients.

5. In many circumstances "respect for autonomy" simply will not arise as a primary issue—for example, dialogue aimed simply at getting more information or clinical encounters that do not involve PSR matters.

6. See Levi (1996).

7. See DeGrazia (1992).

8. As described by Albert Jonsen and Stephen Toulmin (1988), casuistry involves identifying paradigm cases from which moral maxims can be drawn and constructing cumulative arguments that use analogy to extend the applicability of a given maxim (with greater or lesser probability) to a previously unanalyzed moral conflict. The idea is that there are certain cases about whose resolution we can be sure, and that with attention to circumstances we can discern cases that are sufficiently similar so as to fall under the same maxim. From the Latin, meaning "compendiums," *summae* are collections of philosophical and religious opinions characteristic of the casuistic method and were intended to establish canons for the conceptual analysis of everything from the moral life to the nature of the universe. These sorts of "investigations" actually antedate casuistry by a few hundred years, with notable works including Peter Abelard's *Theology of the Supreme Good* (circa 1130) and Thomas Aquinas's *Summa Theologica* (1272).

9. "House-keeping issues" is a term used by Virginia Warren (1989) to shift our ethical focus away from competitive power struggles with their narrow range of alternative actions to a larger reassessment of the structure of our interactions, how we think about ourselves, and specifically how we relate to others.

10. So, for example, when Sally decides to get her fallopian tubes tied, it would be an empirical matter that this decision involves her husband, probably her par-

ents and in-laws, perhaps her estranged brother, most likely not her newspaper delivery girl, and almost certainly not someone halfway across the world who is entirely unaware of Sally's existence.

11. Because the strong relationist claim relies on personal rather than contractual relationships, neither financial matters (e.g., who owns the house they live in) nor service arrangements (e.g., does May "do" more for Leo, or vice versa) should make much difference for the issue being addressed here.

12. There are, in fact, many further aspects of this argument that merit exploring, but I fear they would become rather involved and would detract from the overall line of argument I wish to pursue.

13. A related concern that is not necessarily an objection is as follows. If indeed membership in a relationship is what is pivotal about whether or not one has a role in a decision-making process, does this mean that for everyone sufficiently proximately related there is an attendant responsibility to play a role in the decision-making process?

14. For example, respect for autonomy entails (to a greater or lesser extent) the atomistic view that it makes sense to subdivide human society into individual units, along with the assumption that individuals should be understood as the authors of their lives. Given the influence of language and culture, as well as institutional frameworks within society, baggage such as this at times may prove burdensome to carry.

15. Specifically, developing more substantive relationships with patients has been shown to increase diagnostic accuracy and therapeutic outcomes (see Korsch, Gozzi, and Francis 1968; Francis, Korsch, and Morris 1969; Waitzkin and Stoeckle 1972; Frankel and Beckstein 1982; Goldberg et al. 1980) as well as decrease litigation costs, the incidence of malpractice suits, and the excessive use of expensive diagnostic and therapeutic technologies (see Charles 1992; Westman, Lewandoski, and Proctor 1993).

16. Because intimacy may be defined in varying ways, not all forms of intimacy, of course, will depend upon the existence of a deep and lasting relationship. Sometimes it is easier to be intimate precisely because the other person is an absolute stranger. Also, various professional boundaries in and of themselves may facilitate intimacy insofar as they assuage people's sense of vulnerability.

17. I say *reasonable* because it is inappropriate to expect HCPs to do everything possible to benefit their patients' health.

18. See, for example, the President's Commission for the Study of Ethical Problems in Medicine and Biomedical and Behavioral Research (1983). The distinction between demands for noninterference versus demands for aid is itself a matter of serious philosophical discussion. See Berlin (1969).

19. Clarifying this issue in part will involve trying to distinguish HCPs' professional judgments about the right thing to do in a particular circumstance from their personal judgments. So, for example, it would be important to distinguish the medical judgment that circumcision of a male infant is unwarranted from the per-

sonal judgment that it is unwarranted. Obviously, how to make such distinctions quickly becomes an extremely complex issue. For one approach to dealing with this issue, see Gert, Bernat, and Mogielnicki (1994).

20. Obviously, which health care services would be guaranteed would vary depending on society's conception of what it is reasonable to expect. Still, "to claim to guarantee people a right that they are in fact unable to exercise is fraudulent, like furnishing people with meal tickets but providing no food" (Shue 1980:27).

21. See Bruce Vladeck (1980:19) for this account and a more general discussion of this issue. Other discussions that evidence the absence of substantive change since Vladeck's insightful analysis include Dodds (1996); Gamroth, Semradeck, and Tornquist (1995); and Olsen, Chichin, and Libow (1995).

22. *Pro re nata* = according to circumstances, i.e., as needed.

Chapter 8: A Brief Assessment of the Model

1. A particularly influential program based on this premise is Stephen Covey's *Seven Habits of Highly Effective People* (1989). In its essence, the Covey program calls on each individual to infuse her core principles into her everyday habits, and in doing so work to build relationships with others based on trust and respect.

2. See Arnold (1993); Friedman and Mennin (1991); Monahan et al. (1988); Stemmler (1986); and Robert Smith (1984).

3. This unpublished study was conducted during the spring of 1996 at the University of Illinois as part of the introduction to clinical medicine portion of the second-year curriculum. Students in the experimental group received seven hours of lecture-discussion on the concept of autonomy, exploring what autonomy is and what it might mean to respect patients' autonomous PSR decisions. Students in the control group also received seven hours of lecture-discussion, but their curriculum dealt with a general set of bioethics-related concerns, such as the effect of managed care on the practice of medicine, professional expectations of physicians, and the doctor-nurse relationship. Though substantially altered, the format used for evaluating the students borrowed significantly from the University of Toronto model for ethics OSCEs developed by Peter Singer et al. (1994).

4. For example, a nurse might explain to a family member that despite the patient's clearly expressed advance directives, there is no do not resuscitate order on the chart because the physician has not written it. The nurse might even explain that she does not feel comfortable confronting the physician about the omission since hospital policy generally is not supportive of nurses in such situations. An HCP might admit to the patient that the reason an extended appointment is not possible is because the HMO will not reimburse primary care practitioners for counseling and that practitioners must meet a production quota to keep their jobs. It is honesty more than courage or a willingness to be confrontational that is at issue here—honesty about why what should be done is not being done.

Bibliography

Abernethy, Virginia. 1991. "Judgments about Patient Competence: Cultural and Economic Antecedents." In *Competency: A Study of Informal Competency Determinations in Primary Care,* ed. Mary Ann Cutter and Earl Shelp. Dordrecht, the Netherlands: Kluwer Academic Publishers. 211–27.

Allen, R. T. 1982. "Rational Autonomy: The Destruction of Freedom." *Journal of Philosophy of Education* 16 (2): 199–207.

Almond, Brenda. 1988. "Women's Right: Reflections on Ethics and Gender." In *Feminist Perspectives in Philosophy,* ed. Morwenna Griffiths and Margaret Whitford. Bloomington: Indiana University Press. 42–57.

Appelbaum, Paul, and Thomas Grisso. 1988. "Assessing Patients' Capacities to Consent to Treatment." *New England Journal of Medicine* 319 (25): 1635–38.

Arneson, Richard. 1991. "Autonomy and Preference Formation." Ms.

Arnold, Robert. 1993. "Assessing Competence in Clinical Ethics." *Journal of General Internal Medicine* 8 (Jan.): 52–54.

Arras, John. 1991. "Getting Down to Cases: The Revival of Casuistry in Bioethics." *Journal of Medicine and Philosophy* 16 (1): 29–51.

Arras, John, and Nancy Rhoden, eds. 1989. *Ethical Issues in Modern Medicine.* 3d ed. Mountain View, Calif.: Mayfield.

Barclay, Mel, and Thomas Elkins. 1991. "A Computer Conference Format for Teaching Medical Ethics." *Academic Medicine* 66 (10): 592–94.

Battin, Margaret. 1991. "The Least Worst Death." In *Biomedical Ethics,* ed. Thomas A. Mappes and Jane S. Zembaty. 3d ed. New York: McGraw-Hill. 336–41.

Beauchamp, Thomas. 1991. "Competence." In *Competency: A Study of Informal Competency Determinations in Primary Care,* ed. Mary Ann Cutter and Earl Shelp. Dordrecht, the Netherlands: Kluwer Academic Publishers. 49–78.

———. 1995. "Principlism and Its Alleged Competitors." *Kennedy Institute of Ethics Journal* 5 (3): 181–98.

Beauchamp, Thomas, and James Childress. 1994. *Principles of Biomedical Ethics.* 4th ed. New York: Oxford University Press.

Beauchamp, Thomas, and Leroy Walters, eds. 1982. *Contemporary Issues in Bioethics.* 2d ed. Belmont, Calif.: Wadsworth.

Benhabib, Seyla. 1987. "The Generalized and Concrete Other." In *Women and Moral Theory,* ed. Diana Meyers and E. F. Kittay. Totawa, N.J.: Rowman and Littlefield. 154–77.

Benn, Stanley. 1976. "Freedom, Autonomy, and the Concept of a Person." *Proceedings of the Aristotelian Society* 12 (76): 109–30.

———. 1982. "Individuality, Autonomy, and Community." In *Community as a Social Ideal*, ed. E. Kamenka. London: E. Arnold. 43–62.

———. 1988. *A Theory of Freedom*. New York: Cambridge University Press.

Berlin, Isaiah. 1969. *Four Essays on Liberty*. New York: Oxford University Press.

Bernstein, Richard. 1991. *Beyond Objectivism and Relativism: Science, Hermeneutics, and Praxis*. Philadelphia: University of Pennsylvania Press.

Berofsky, Bernard. 1995. *Liberation from Self: A Theory of Personal Autonomy*. New York: Cambridge University Press.

Bickel, Janet. 1987. "Human Values Teaching Programs in the Clinical Education of Medical Students." *Journal of Medical Education* 62 (May): 369–78.

———. 1991. "Medical Students' Professional Ethics: Defining the Problems and Developing Resources." *Academic Medicine* 66 (12): 726–29.

Blake, C., and J. M. Morfitt. 1986. "Falls and Staffing in a Residential Home for Elderly People." *Public Health* 100:385–91.

Blakeslee, Jill. 1988. "Untie the Elderly." *American Journal of Nursing* 88 (6): 833–34.

Blustein, Jeffrey. 1993. "The Family in Medical Decisionmaking." *Hastings Center Report* 23 (3): 6–13.

Boller, Paul. 1977. "Freedom in John Dewey's Philosophy of Education." *Teachers College Record* 79 (1): 99–118.

Brandt, Richard. 1979. *A Theory of the Good and the Right*. New York: Oxford University Press.

Bresnahan, James. 1988. "Paternalism and Autonomy." *Ethics* 99 (3): 551–65.

Bresnahan, James, and Kathryn Hunter. 1989. "Ethics Education at Northwestern University Medical School." *Academic Medicine* 64 (12): 740–44.

Bresnahan, James, and Steven Whartman. 1990. "When Competent Patients Make Irrational Choices." *New England Journal of Medicine* 322 (22): 1595–99.

Buchanan, Allen. 1978. "Medical Paternalism." *Philosophy and Public Affairs* 7 (4): 371–90.

Burbules, Nicholas. 1993. *Dialogue in Teaching: Theory and Practice*. New York: Teachers College Press.

Callahan, Daniel. 1996. "Can the Moral Commons Survive Autonomy?" *Hastings Center Report* 26 (6): 41–42.

Callan, Eamonn. 1988. *Autonomy and Schooling*. Montreal: McGill-Queen's University Press.

Carse, Alisa. 1991. "The 'Voice of Care': Implications for Bioethical Education." *Journal of Medicine and Philosophy* 16 (1): 5–28.

Carse, Alisa, and H. L. Nelson. 1996. "Rehabilitating Care." *Kennedy Institute of Ethics Journal* 6 (1): 19–36.

Charles, S. C. 1992. "Predicting Risk for Medical Malpractice Claims Using Quality-of-Care Characteristics." *Western Journal of Medicine* 157 (4): 433–39.

Childress, James. 1983. *Who Should Decide?: Paternalism in Healthcare.* New York: Oxford University Press.

———. 1990. "The Place of Autonomy in Bioethics." *Hastings Center Report* 20 (1): 12–17.

Childress, James, and John C. Fletcher. 1994. "Respect for Autonomy." *Hastings Center Report* 24 (3): 34–35.

Christman, John. 1987. "Autonomy: A Defense of the Split-Level Self." *Southern Journal of Philosophy* 25 (3): 281–93.

———. 1988. "Constructing the Inner Citadel: Recent Work on the Concept of Autonomy." *Ethics* 99 (1): 109–21.

———, ed. 1989. *The Inner Citadel: Essays on Individual Autonomy.* New York: Oxford University Press.

Clement, Grace. 1996. *Care, Autonomy, and Justice: Feminism and the Ethic of Care.* Boulder: Westview Press.

Clouser, K. Danner, and Bernard Gert. 1990. "A Critique of Principlism." *Journal of Medicine and Philosophy* 15 (2): 219–36.

Cohen, Robert. 1991. "Assessing Competency to Address Ethical Issues in Medicine." *Academic Medicine* 66 (1): 14–15.

Colby, Kathleen, Thomas Almy, and Michael Zubkoff. 1986. "Problem-Based Learning of Social Sciences and Humanities by Fourth-Year Medical Students." *Journal of Medical Education* 61 (May): 413–15.

Covert, Anthony, Theresa Rodrigues, and Kenneth Solomon. 1977. "The Use of Mechanical and Chemical Restraints in Nursing Homes." *Journal of the American Geriatrics Society* 25 (2): 85–89.

Covey, Stephen. 1989. *Seven Habits of Highly Effective People.* New York: Simon and Schuster.

Crapanzano, Vincent. 1990. "On Dialogue." In *The Interpretation of Dialogue,* ed. Tullio Maranhao. Chicago: University of Chicago Press. 262–91.

Culver, Charles, and Bernard Gert. 1982. *Philosophy in Medicine.* New York: Oxford University Press.

Cutter, Mary Ann, and Earl Shelp, eds. 1991. *Competency: A Study of Informal Competency Determinations in Primary Care.* Dordrecht, the Netherlands: Kluwer Academic Publishers.

Daelemans, Sven, and Tullio Maranhao. 1990. "Psychoanalytic Dialogue and the Dialogical Principle." In *The Interpretation of Dialogue,* ed. Tullio Maranhao. Chicago: University of Chicago Press. 219–41.

Daniels, Norman. 1979. "Wide Reflective Equilibrium and Theory Acceptance in Ethics." *Journal of Philosophy* 76 (56): 257–73.

———. 1980. "Reflective Equilibrium and Archimedean Points." *Canadian Journal of Philosophy* 10 (1): 83–103.

Davis, Dena. 1986. "Am I My Doppelganger's Keeper?: Autonomy, Paternalism, and Authentic Decision-Making." Ph.D. diss., University of Iowa.

DeGrazia, David. 1992. "Moving Forward in Bioethical Theory: Theories, Cases, and Specified Principlism." *Journal of Medicine and Philosophy* 17 (5): 511–39.

Dewey, John. 1957. *Human Nature and Conduct.* New York: Modern Library.

———. 1987. *Experience and Nature.* La Salle, Ill.: Open Court Classics.

Dixon, Kathleen. 1985. "Paternalism and Autonomy." Ph.D. diss., University of Tennessee.

Dodds, Susan. 1996. "Exercising Restraint: Autonomy, Welfare, and Elerly Patients." *Journal of Medical Ethics* 22 (3): 160–63.

Downie, R. S., and Elizabeth Tefler. 1971. "Autonomy." *Philosophy* 46 (178): 293–301.

Dresser, Rebecca, and P. J. Whitehouse. 1994. "The Incompetent Patient on the Slippery Slope." *Hastings Center Report* 24 (4): 6–12.

Dubose, Edwin, Jr., and Earl Shelp. 1991. "Competency Judgments: Case Studies in Moral Perspective." In *Competency: A Study of Informal Competency Determinations in Primary Care,* ed. Mary Ann Cutter and Earl Shelp. Dordrecht, the Netherlands: Kluwer Academic Publishers. 185–93.

Dworkin, Gerald. 1988. *The Theory and Practice of Autonomy.* New York: Cambridge University Press.

Dworkin, Ronald. 1978. *Taking Rights Seriously.* Cambridge: Harvard University Press.

Edwards, Rem B. 1981. "Mental Health as Rational Autonomy." *Journal of Medicine and Philosophy* 6 (3): 309–22.

Edwards, Rem B., and Thomas Szasz, eds. 1997. *Ethics of Psychiatry: Insanity, Rational Autonomy, and Mental Health Care.* Boston: Prometheus Books.

Elkins, Thomas. 1988. "Introductory Course in Biomedical Ethics in the Obstetrics-Gynecology Residency." *Journal of Medical Education* 63:294–300.

Elliott, Carl. 1992. "Where Ethics Comes From and What to Do about It." *Hastings Center Report* 22 (4): 28–35.

Ellul, Jacques. 1973. *Propaganda: The Formation of Men's Attitudes.* New York: Vintage Books.

Elster, Jon. 1982. "Sour Grapes: Utilitarianism and the Genesis of Wants." In *Utilitarianism and Beyond,* ed. Amartya Sen and Bernard Williams. Cambridge: Cambridge University Press. 219–32.

Ende, Jack, Lewis Kazis, Arlene Ash, and Mark A. Moskowitz. 1989. "Measuring Patients' Desire for Autonomy." *Journal of General Internal Medicine* 4 (Jan.–Feb.): 23–29.

Engelhardt, Tristram. 1986. *The Foundations of Bioethics.* New York: Oxford University Press.

Erde, Edmund. 1991. "Breaking Up the Shell Game of Consequentialism: Incompetence—Concept and Ethics." *Competency: A Study of Informal Competency Determinations in Primary Care,* ed. Mary Ann Cutter and Earl Shelp. Dordrecht, the Netherlands: Kluwer Academic Publishers. 237–52.

Evans, Lois, and Neville Strumpf. 1989. "Tying Down the Elderly: A Review of the

Literature on Physical Restraint." *Journal of the American Geriatric Society* 37 (Jan.): 65–74.

Feinberg, Joel. 1973. *Social Philosophy*. Englewood Cliffs, N.J.: Prentice Hall.

————. 1980. "The Child's Right to an Open Future." In *Whose Child?: Children's Rights, Parental Authority, and State Power,* ed. William Aiken and Hugh LaFollette. Totowa, N.J.: Rowman and Littlefield. 124–53.

————. 1986. *Harm to Self*. New York: Oxford University Press.

Ferrara, Alessandro. 1990. "A Critique of Habermas's Diskusethik." In *The Interpretation of Dialogue,* ed. Tullio Maranhao. Chicago: University of Chicago Press. 303–37.

Forrow, Lachlan, Robert Arnold, and Joel Frader. 1991. "Teaching Clinical Ethics in the Residency Years: Preparing Competent Professionals." *Journal of Medicine and Philosophy* 16 (1): 93–112.

Fox-Genovese, Elizabeth. 1991. *Feminism without Illusions*. Chapel Hill: University of North Carolina Press.

Francis, V., B. M. Korsch, and M. J. Morris. 1969. "Gaps in Doctor-Patient Communication: Patients' Responses to Medical Advice." *New England Journal of Medicine* 280 (10): 535–40.

Frankel, R. M., and H. A. Beckstein. 1982. *Impact: An Interaction-Based Method in Explorations in Provider and Patient Interactions*. Clifton, N.J.: Humana Press.

Frankena, William. 1973. *Ethics*. 2d ed. New York: Prentice Hall.

Frankfurt, Harry. 1971. "Freedom of the Will and the Concept of a Person." *Journal of Philosophy* 68 (1): 5–20.

Friedman, Marilyn. 1989. "Self-Rule in Social Context: Autonomy from a Feminist Perspective." In *Freedom, Equality, and Social Change,* ed. Creighton Peden and James Sterba. Lewiston, N.Y.: Edwin Mellen Press. 158–69.

Friedman, Miriam, and Stewart Mennin. 1991. "Rethinking Critical Issues in Performance Assessment." *Academic Medicine* 66 (7): 390–96.

Gamroth, Lucia, Joyce Semradeck, and Elizabeth M. Tornquist. 1995. *Enhancing Autonomy in Long Term Care: Concepts and Strategies*. New York: Springer.

Gaylin, Willard. 1996. "Worshipping Autonomy." *Hastings Center Report* 26 (6): 43–45.

Gaylin, Willard, and Bruce Jennings. 1996. *The Perversion of Autonomy*. New York: Free Press.

Gert, Bernard. 1973. *The Moral Rules*. New York: Harper and Row.

Gert, Bernard, J. L. Bernat, and R. P. Mogielnicki. 1994. "Distinguishing between Patients' Refusals and Requests." *Hastings Center Report* 24 (4): 13–15.

Gert, Bernard, and K. Danner Clouser. 1986. "Rationality in Medicine: An Explication." *Journal of Medicine and Philosophy* 11 (3): 185–205.

Gert, Bernard, and Charles Culver. 1982. *Philosophy in Medicine*. New York: Oxford University Press.

Gert, Bernard, and Timothy Duggan. 1979. "Free Will as the Ability to Will." *Nous* 13 (2): 197–217.

Gibson, Mary. 1977. "Rationality." *Philosophy and Public Affairs* 6 (3): 193–225.

Gilligan, Carol. 1982. "In a Different Voice: Women's Conceptions of Self and of Morality." *Harvard Educational Review* 47 (4): 481–517.

———. 1987. "Moral Orientation and Moral Development." In *Women and Moral Theory,* ed. Diana Meyers and E. F. Kittay. Totawa, N.J.: Rowman and Littlefield. 19–33.

Gillon, Raanan. 1985. "Autonomy and Consent." In *Moral Dilemmas in Modern Medicine,* ed. Michael Lockwood. New York: Oxford University Press. 111–25.

Goldberg, D. P., J. J. Steele, C. Smith, and L. Spivey. 1980. "Training Family Doctors to Recognise Psychiatric Illness with Increased Accuracy." *Lancet* 2 (8193): 521–23.

Goodin, Robert. 1985. *Protecting the Vulnerable.* Chicago: University of Chicago Press.

Green, Ronald. 1990. "Method in Bioethics: A Troubled Assessment." *Journal of Medicine and Philosophy* 15 (2): 179–97.

Grimshaw, Jean. 1988. "Autonomy and Identity in Feminist Thinking." In *Feminist Perspectives in Philosophy,* ed. Morwenna Griffiths and Margaret Whitford. Bloomington: Indiana University Press. 91–108.

Gustafson, James. 1990. "Moral Discourse about Medicine: A Variety of Forms." *Journal of Medicine and Philosophy* 15 (5): 125–42.

Habermas, Jürgen. 1984. *Theory of Communicative Action.* Boston: Beacon Press.

Halper, Thomas. 1980. "The Double-Edged Sword: Paternalism as a Policy in the Problems of Aging." *Milbank Memorial Fund Quarterly/Health and Society* 58 (3): 199–226.

———. 1996. "Privacy and Autonomy: From Warren and Brandeis to *Roe* and *Cruzan.*" *Journal of Medicine and Philosophy* 21 (2): 121–35.

Hamilton, Edith, and Huntington Cairns, eds. 1989. *Plato: The Collected Dialogues.* Princeton: Princeton University Press.

Hart, Herbert Lionel Adolphus. 1955. "Are There Any Natural Rights." *Philosophical Review* 64 (2): 175–91.

Haworth, Lawrence. 1986. *Autonomy.* New Haven: Yale University Press.

Hendrie, Hugh, and Camille Lloyd, eds. 1990. *Educating Competent and Human Physicians.* Bloomington: Indiana University Press.

Hershey, Paul. 1985. "A Definition for Paternalism." *Journal of Medicine and Philosophy* 10 (2): 171–82.

High, Dallas. 1989. "Caring for Decisionally Incapacitated Elderly." *Theoretical Medicine* 10:83–96.

Hill, Thomas. 1987. "The Importance of Autonomy." In *Women and Moral Theory,* ed. Diana Meyers and E. F. Kittay. Totawa, N.J.: Rowman and Littlefield. 129–38.

Hing, Esther. 1987. "Use of Nursing Homes by the Elderly: Preliminary Data from the 1985 National Nursing Home Survey." *Advanced Data* 135 (May): 1–11.

Holmes, Robert. 1990. "The Limited Relevance of Analytic Ethics to the Problems of Bioethics." *Journal of Medicine and Philosophy* 15 (2): 143–59.

Hughes, Judith. 1988. "The Philosopher's Child." In *Feminist Perspectives in Philosophy,* ed. Morwenna Griffiths and Margaret Whitford. Bloomington: Indiana University Press. 72–89.

Humphrey, Derek. 1991. *Final Exit.* Eugene, Ore.: Hemlock Society.

Hurka, Thomas. 1987. "Why Value Autonomy?" *Social Theory and Practice* 13 (3): 361–82.

Husak, Douglas. 1980. "Paternalism and Autonomy." *Philosophy and Public Affairs* 10 (1): 27–46.

Huyssen, Andreas. 1990. "Mapping the Postmodern." In *Feminism/Postmodernism,* ed. Linda Nicholson. New York: Routledge. 234–77.

Jonsen, Albert. 1990. *The New Medicine and the Old Ethics.* Cambridge, Mass.: Harvard University Press.

———. 1991. "American Moralism and the Origin of Bioethics in the United States." *Journal of Medicine and Philosophy* 16 (1): 113–30.

Jonsen, Albert, Mark Siegler, and William Winslade. 1992. *Clinical Ethics.* 3d ed. New York: McGraw-Hill.

Jonsen, Albert, and Stephen Toulmin. 1988. *The Abuse of Casuistry.* Berkeley: University of California Press.

Kapp, Marshall. 1988. *Legal Aspects of Health Care for the Elderly: An Annotated Bibliography.* New York: Greenwood Press.

———. 1989. "Medical Empowerment of the Elderly." *Hastings Center Report* 19 (4): 5–7.

Kleinig, John. 1984. *Paternalism.* Totowa, N.J.: Rowman and Allanheld.

Kliever, Lonnie, ed. 1991. *Dax's Case: Essays in Medical Ethics and Human Meaning.* Dallas: Southern Methodist University Press.

Knight, James. 1991. "Judging Competence: When the Psychiatrist Need, or Need Not, Be Involved." In *Competency: A Study of Informal Competency Determinations in Primary Care,* ed. Mary Ann Cutter and Earl Shelp. Dordrecht, the Netherlands: Kluwer Academic Publishers. 3–28.

Kopelman, Loretta. 1990. "What Is Applied about Applied Philosophy?" *Journal of Medicine and Philosophy* 15 (2): 199–218.

Korsch, B. M., E. K. Gozzi, and V. Francis. 1968. "Gaps in Doctor-Patient Communication: Doctor-Patient Interaction and Patient Satisfaction." *Pediatrics* 42 (5): 855–71.

Kuhn, Thomas. 1970. *The Structure of Scientific Revolutions.* 2d ed., enl. Chicago: University of Chicago Press.

Ladenson, Robert. 1975. "A Theory of Personal Autonomy." *Ethics* 86 (1): 30–48.

Lamb, Karen, Joanne Miller, and Margaret Hernandez. 1987. "Falls in the Elderly: Causes and Prevention." *Orthopaedic Nursing* 6 (2): 45–49.

Laor, Nathaniel. 1984. "The Paradox of Autonomy: The Case of the Mentally Ill." *Journal of Value Inquiry* 18 (2): 159–66.

Levi, Benjamin. 1996. "Four Approaches to Doing Ethics." *Journal of Medicine and Philosophy* 21 (1): 7–39.

Lidz, Charles, Lynn Fischer, and Robert Arnold. 1992. *The Erosion of Autonomy in Long-Term Care.* New York: Oxford University Press.

Little, Margaret Olivia. 1996. "Why a Feminist Approach to Bioethics." *Kennedy Institute of Ethics Journal* 6 (1): 1–18.

Loewy, Erich. 1986. "Teaching Medical Ethics to Medical Students." *Journal of Medical Education* 61 (8): 661–65.

Lustig, B. Andrew. 1992. "The Method of 'Principlism': A Critique of the Critique." *Journal of Medicine and Philosophy* 17 (5): 487–510.

MacCallum, Gerald. 1967. "Negative and Positive Freedom." *Philosophical Review* 76 (3): 312–34.

MacIntyre, Alisdair. 1984. *After Virtue.* 2d ed. Notre Dame: University of Notre Dame Press.

Mahowald, Mary. 1995. "Person." In *Encyclopedia of Bioethics,* ed. Warren T. Reich. New York: Macmillan. 1934–40.

Mappes, Thomas A., and Jane S. Zembaty, eds. 1991. *Biomedical Ethics.* 3d ed. New York: McGraw-Hill.

Maranhao, Tullio, ed. 1990. *The Interpretation of Dialogue.* Chicago: University of Chicago Press.

Martin, Michael. 1986. "Defining Irrational Action in Medical and Psychiatric Contexts." *Journal of Medicine and Philosophy* 11 (2): 179–84.

McDonald, Michael. 1978. "Autarchy and Interest." *Australasian Journal of Philosophy* 56 (2): 109–25.

McIninch, Amy. 1989. "The Case Method in Teacher Education: Analysis, Rationale, and Proposal." Ph.D. diss., University of Illinois.

McKnight, Christopher J. 1993. "Autonomy and the Akratic Patient." *Journal of Medical Ethics* 19 (4): 206–10.

Meyers, Diana. 1987. "Personal Autonomy and the Paradox of Feminine Socialization." *Journal of Philosophy* 84 (11): 619–28.

Miles, Steven, Laura Weiss Lane, Janet Bickel, Robert M. Walker, and Christine K. Cassel. 1989. "Medical Ethics Education: Coming of Age." *Academic Medicine* 64 (12): 705–15.

Mill, John Stuart. 1947. *On Liberty.* New York: Appleton-Century-Crofts.

Misik, Irene. 1981. "About Using Restraints—With Restraint." *Nursing* 11 (Aug.): 50–55.

Mitchell, Christine. 1986. "Code Grey: Considering the Principle of Autonomy." *Nursing Life* (Mar.–Apr.): 26–30.

Monahan, Deborah, P. L. Grover, R. E. Kavey, J. L. Greenwald, E. C. Jacobsen, and H. L. Weinberger. 1988. "Evaluation of a Communication Skills Course for Second-Year Medical Students." *Journal of Medical Education* 63 (5): 372–78.

Moody, Thomas. 1989. "Liberal Conceptions of the Self and Autonomy." In *Freedom, Equality, and Social Change,* ed. Creighton Peden and James Sterba. Lewiston, N.Y.: Edwin Mellen Press. 94–108.

Morreim, Haavi. 1991. "Competence: At the Intersection of Law, Medicine, and

Philosophy." In *Competency: A Study of Informal Competency Determinations in Primary Care,* ed. Mary Ann Cutter and Earl Shelp. Dordrecht, the Netherlands: Kluwer Academic Publishers. 93–126.

Moskowitz, Ellen H. 1996. "Moral Consensus in Public Ethics: Patient Autonomy and Family Decisionmaking in the Work of One State Bioethics Commission." *Journal of Medicine and Philosophy* 21 (2): 149–68.

Murray, Thomas H. 1994. "Communities Need More than Autonomy." *Hastings Center Report* 24 (3): 32–33.

Neely, Wright. 1974. "Freedom and Desire." *Philosophical Review* 83 (1): 32–54.

Okin, Susan. 1991. *Justice, Gender, and the Family.* New York: Basic Books.

Olsen, Ellen, Eileen Chichin, and Leslie Libow, eds. 1995. *Controversies in Ethics in Long Term Care.* New York: Springer.

O'Neill, Onora. 1984. "Paternalism and Partial Autonomy." *Journal of Medical Ethics* 10 (4): 173–78.

Parfit, Derek. 1986. *Reasons and Persons.* New York: Oxford University Press.

Pellegrino, Edmund. 1991. "Informal Judgments of Competence and Incompetence." In *Competency: A Study of Informal Competency Determinations in Primary Care,* ed. Mary Ann Cutter and Earl Shelp. Dordrecht, the Netherlands: Kluwer Academic Publishers. 29–45.

Perl, Mark. 1991. "Competency Judgments: Case Studies from the Psychiatrist's Perspective." In *Competency: A Study of Informal Competency Determinations in Primary Care,* ed. Mary Ann Cutter and Earl Shelp. Dordrecht, the Netherlands: Kluwer Academic Publishers. 179–84.

Peters, Richard S. 1967. "Hobbes, Thomas." In *The Encyclopedia of Philosophy,* ed. Paul Edwards. New York: Macmillan. 30–46.

Pincoffs, Edmund. 1991. "Judgments of Incompetence and Their Moral Presuppositions." In *Competency: A Study of Informal Competency Determinations in Primary Care,* ed. Mary Ann Cutter and Earl Shelp. Dordrecht, the Netherlands: Kluwer Academic Publishers. 79–89.

President's Commission for the Study of Ethical Problems in Medicine and Biomedical and Behavioral Research. 1983. *Deciding to Forego Life-Sustaining Treatment: A Report on the Ethical, Medical, and Legal Issues in Treatment Decisions.* Washington, D.C.: U.S. Government Printing Office.

Puckett, Andrew, D. G. Graham, L. A. Pound, and F. T. Nash. 1989. "The Duke University Program for Integrating Ethics and Human Values into Medical Education." *Academic Medicine* 64 (5): 231–35.

Quine, Willard. 1951. "Two Dogmas of Empiricism." *Philosophical Review* 60 (1): 20–43.

Quill, Timothy, and Howard Brody. 1996. "Physician Recommendations and Patient Autonomy: Finding a Balance." *Annals of Internal Medicine* 125 (9): 763–69.

Radwany, Steven, and Bernard Adelson. 1987. "The Use of Literary Classics in Teaching Medical Ethics to Physicians." *Journal of the American Medical Association* 257 (12): 1629–31.

Rawls, John. 1971. *A Theory of Justice.* Cambridge, Mass.: Harvard University Press.

———. 1980. "Kantian Constructivism in Moral Theory: Rational and Full Autonomy." *Journal of Philosophy* 77 (9): 515–35.

Redmon, Robert. 1989. "A Medical Ethics Project for Third-Year Medical Students." *Academic Medicine* 64 (5): 266–70.

Rhymes, Jill. 1987. "Autonomy and Decision Making for Nursing Home Residents." Ms.

Richards, David. 1981. "Rights and Autonomy." *Ethics* 92 (1): 3–20.

Richardson, Henry. 1990. "Specifying Norms as a Way to Resolve Concrete Ethical Problems." *Philosophy and Public Affairs* 19 (3): 279–310.

Robbins, Laurence, Edward Boyko, Judy Lane, Darcy Cooper, and Dennis W. Jahnigen. 1987. "Binding the Elderly: A Prospective Study in the Use of Mechanical Restraints in an Acute Care Hospital." *Journal of the American Geriatrics Society* 35 (4): 290–96.

Roth, Loren, Alan Meisel, and Charles Lidz. 1977. "Tests of Competency to Consent to Treatment." *American Journal of Psychiatry* 134 (3): 279–84.

Rothman, David. 1991. *Strangers at the Bedside: A History of How Law and Bioethics Transformed Medical Decision Making.* New York: Basic Books.

Ryden, Muriel. 1985. "Environmental Support for Autonomy in the Institutionalized Elderly." *Research in Nursing and Health* 8 (Sept.): 363–71.

Sankowski, Edward. 1985. "Paternalism and Social Policy." *American Philosophical Quarterly* 22 (1): 1–12.

———. 1989. "Some Problems about One Liberal Conception of Autonomy." *Australasian Journal of Philosophy* 67 (3): 277–85.

Sartorius, Rolf. 1983. *Paternalism.* Minneapolis: University of Minnesota Press.

Schafer, Arthur. 1985. "Restraints and the Elderly: When Safety and Autonomy Conflict." *Canadian Medical Association Journal* 132 (June): 1257–60.

Schaffner, Kenneth. 1991. "Competency: A Triaxial Concept." In *Competency: A Study of Informal Competency Determinations in Primary Care,* ed. Mary Ann Cutter and Earl Shelp. Dordrecht, the Netherlands: Kluwer Academic Publishers. 253–81.

Scoccia, Danny. 1987. "Autonomy, Want Satisfaction, and the Justification of Liberal Freedoms." *Canadian Journal of Philosophy* 17 (3): 583–602.

———. 1990. "Paternalism and Respect for Autonomy." *Ethics* 100 (2): 318–34.

Scully, Thomas, and Celia Scully. 1987. *Playing God: The New World of Medical Choices.* New York: Simon and Schuster.

Shapiro, Ian. 1988. *The Evolution of Rights in Liberal Theory.* Cambridge: Cambridge University Press.

Sherwin, Susan. 1989. "Feminist and Medical Ethics: Two Different Approaches to Contextual Ethics." *Hypatia* 4 (2): 52–72.

———. 1992. *No Longer Patient.* Philadelphia: Temple University Press.

Shue, Henry. 1980. *Basic Rights.* Princeton: Princeton University Press.

Siegler, Mark. 1985. "The Progression of Medicine: From Physician Paternalism to

Patient Autonomy to Bureaucratic Parsimony." *Archives of Internal Medicine* 145 (Apr.): 713–15.

Singer, Peter, A. Robb, R. Cohen, G. Norman, and J. Turnbull. 1994. "Evaluation of a Multicenter Ethics Objective Structured Clinical Examination." *Journal of General Internal Medicine* 9 (Dec.): 690–92.

Smith, George. 1995. *Liberation from Self: A Theory of Personal Autonomy.* Cambridge: Cambridge University Press.

Smith, Janet Farrel. 1996. "Communicative Ethics in Medicine: The Physician-Patient Relationship." In *Feminism and Bioethics,* ed. Susan Wolf. New York: Oxford University Press. 184–215.

Smith, Robert. 1984. "Teaching Interviewing Skills to Medical Students: The Issue of Countertransference." *Journal of Medical Education* 59 (7): 582–88.

Soble, Alan. 1982. "Paternalism, Liberal Theory, and Suicide." *Canadian Journal of Philosophy* 12 (2): 335–52.

Stemmler, Edward. 1986. "Promoting Improved Evaluation of Students during Clinical Education: A Complex Management Task." *Journal of Medical Education* 61 (suppl.): 75–82.

Strasser, Mark. 1988. "The New Paternalism." *Bioethics* 2 (2): 103–17.

Sunstein, Cass. 1991. "Rightalk." *New Republic,* Sept. 2: 33–36.

Swearingen, Jan. 1990. "Dialogue and Dialectic: The Logic of Conversation and the Interpretation of Logic." In *The Interpretation of Dialogue,* ed. Tullio Maranhao. Chicago: University of Chicago Press. 47–71.

Szasz, Thomas. 1970. *Manufacture of Madness: A Comparative Study of the Inquisition and the Mental Health Movement.* New York: Harper and Row.

Tannsjo, Torbjorn. 1989. "Against Personal Autonomy." *International Journal of Applied Philosophy* (Spring): 45–56.

Taylor, Charles. 1976. "Responsibility for Self." In *The Identity of Persons,* ed. Amelie Rorty. Berkeley: University of California Press. 281–99.

———. 1979. "Atomism." In *Powers, Possessions, and Freedom,* ed. Alkis Kontos. Toronto: University of Toronto Press. 114–34.

Thomas, Dylan. 1953. *The Doctors and the Devils.* New York: James Laughlin Press.

Thomasma, David. 1983. "Beyond Medical Paternalism and Patient Autonomy." *Annals of Internal Medicine* 98 (Feb.): 243–48.

Thomasma, David, and Patricia Marshall. 1989. "The Clinical Medical Humanities Program at Loyola University of Chicago." *Academic Medicine* 64 (12): 735–40.

Thomasma, David, and Edmund Pellegrino. 1988. *For the Patient's Own Good: The Restoration of Beneficence in Health Care.* New York: Oxford University Press.

Thornton, James, and Earl Winkler, eds. 1988. *Ethics and Aging: The Right to Live, the Right to Die.* Vancouver: University of British Columbia Press.

Tibbles, Lance. 1978. "Medical and Legal Aspects of Competency as Affected by Old Age." In *Aging and the Elderly,* ed. Stuart Spicker. Atlantic Highlands, N.J.: Humanities Press. 127–51.

Trilling, Lionel. 1950. *The Liberal Imagination: Essays on Literature and Society.* New York: Viking Press.

Vanderpool, Harold. 1991. "The Competency of Definitions of Competency." In *Competency: A Study of Informal Competency Determinations in Primary Care,* ed. Mary Ann Cutter and Earl Shelp. Dordrecht, the Netherlands: Kluwer Academic Publishers. 197–210.

VanDeVeer, Donald. 1986. *Paternalistic Intervention.* Princeton: Princeton University Press.

Veatch, Robert M. 1995. "Resolving Conflicts among Principles: Ranking, Balancing, and Specifying." *Kennedy Institute of Ethics Journal* 5 (3): 199–218.

————. 1996. "Which Grounds for Overriding Autonomy Are Legitimate?" *Hastings Center Report* 26 (6): 42–43.

Vladeck, Bruce. 1980. *Unloving Care: The Nursing Home Tragedy.* New York: Basic Books.

Waitzkin, Howard, and J. D. Stoeckle. 1972. "The Communication of Information about Illness: Clinical, Sociological, and Methodological Considerations." *Advances in Psychosomatic Medicine* 8:180–215.

Walker, Robert, Laura Lane, and Mark Siegler. 1989. Development of a Teaching Program in Clinical Medical Ethics at the University of Chicago. *Academic Medicine* 64 (12): 723–29.

Warren, Virginia. 1989. "Feminist Directions in Medical Ethics." *Hypatia* 4 (2): 73–87.

Wartman, Steven, and Dan Brock. 1989. "The Development of a Medical Ethics Curriculum in a General Internal Medicine Residency Program." *Academic Medicine* 64 (12): 751–55.

Watson, Gary. 1975. "Free Agency." *Journal of Philosophy* 72 (8): 205–20.

Wear, Stephen. 1991a. "The Irreducibly Clinical Character of Bioethics." *Journal of Medicine and Philosophy* 16 (1): 53–70.

————. 1991b. "Patient Freedom and Competence in Health Care." In *Competency: A Study of Informal Competency Determinations in Primary Care,* ed. Mary Ann Cutter and Earl Shelp. Dordrecht, the Netherlands: Kluwer Academic Publishers. 227–36.

Welie, Jos V. M. 1994. "Authenticity as a Foundational Principle of Medical Ethics." *Theoretical Medicine* 15 (3): 211–15.

Westman, Alida S., Lisa M. Lewandoski, and Susan J. Proctor. 1993. "A Preliminary List to Identify Attitudes toward Different Conditions for Discussing Possible Termination or Refusal of Medical Treatment Except for Pain Relief." *Psychological Reports* 72 (1): 279–84.

White, Betty Cox. 1994. *Competence to Consent.* Washington, D.C.: Georgetown University Press.

White, Morton. 1973. "Positive Freedom, Negative Freedom, and Possibility." *Journal of Philosophy* 70 (11): 309–17.

White, Robert. 1959. "Motivation Reconsidered: The Concept of Competence." *Psychological Review* 66 (5): 297–333.

Wikler, Daniel. 1979. "Paternalism and the Mildly Retarded." *Philosophy and Public Affairs* 8 (4): 377–92.

Wolf, Stewart. 1997. *Educating Doctors: Crisis in Medical Education, Research, and Practice.* New Brunswick, N.J.: Transaction Publishers.

Wolf, Susan. 1992. "Final Exit: The End of Argument." *Hastings Center Report* 22 (1): 30–33.

Wolff, Robert Paul. 1968. *The Poverty of Liberalism.* Boston: Beacon Press.

Wright, Richard. 1991. "Clinical Judgment and Bioethics: The Decision Making Link." *Journal of Medicine and Philosophy* 16 (1): 71–91.

Young, Robert. 1980. "Autonomy and the Inner Self." *American Philosophical Quarterly* 17 (1): 35–43.

———. 1986. *Personal Autonomy: Beyond Negative and Positive Liberty.* New York: St. Martin's Press.

Index

BENJAMIN H. LEVI studied philosophy at Antioch College and St. Andrews University before enrolling in the Medical Scholars Program at the University of Illinois, where he received his M.D. and Ph.D. degrees. Levi has worked as a bioethics consultant and has written several articles on bioethics. He currently works in the Department of Pediatrics at Memorial Medical Center Children's Hospital in Savannah, Georgia.

Typeset in 10.5/13 Minion
with Tekton display
Composed by Barbara Evans
at the University of Illinois Press
Manufactured by Cushing-Malloy, Inc.